HEALTH CARE

OF THE

AGING

HEALTH

CARE

OF THE

AGING

Edited by Harold B. Haley, M.D.,
and Patricia A. Keenan

UNIVERSITY PRESS OF VIRGINIA
Charlottesville

THE UNIVERSITY PRESS OF VIRGINIA
Copyright © 1981 by the Rector and Visitors
of the University of Virginia

First published 1981
The editors and the publisher are grateful for
permission to reprint "Home Style Nursing," by
Mary Kate House, from *Journal of the American
Medical Association*, No. 22, 240 (24 Nov. 1978),
2472-74, copyright 1978, American Medical Association.

Library of Congress Cataloging in Publication Data
Main entry under title:

Health care of the aging.

   Based on papers and panel discussions presented
at two conferences held in 1978 and 1979, sponsored
by the University of Virginia School of Medicine and
the Veterans Administration Medical Center, Salem,
Va.
   Includes bibliographical references and index.
   1. Geriatrics—Congresses.   2. Aged—Care and
hygiene—Congresses.   3. Gerontology—Congresses.
I. Haley, Harold B.   II. Keenan, Patricia A.
III. Virginia.   University.   School of Medicine.
IV. Veterans Administration Medical Center, Salem.
Va. [DNLM: 1. Geriatrics—Congresses.   2. Health
services for the aged—Congresses. WT 30 H4343
1978-79.]   RC952.H39   362.1'9897'0973   80-29409
ISBN 0-8139-0869-8

Printed in the United States of America

To
Norman J. Knorr
without whom we would not have had this book
and
Francis J. Brochu
without whom we would not have had our
Aging and Health Conferences

Contents

Foreword

The University of Virginia School of Medicine is developing
a program in geriatric medicine. Our goal is to improve the
quality of life of the elderly. Our objectives are the
development of research and teaching programs aimed at providing a better understanding of problems concerning the
elderly and the improvement of their health care. Although
patient care is mentioned last, it is understood that only
in the setting where high quality patient care flourishes
can effective research and teaching programs be nourished.
Outlined below is our preliminary thinking related to the
development of our geriatric program.

Should our academic medical center promote the development of specialists in geriatric health care? I think not.
The geriatric program faculty should devote themselves to
an interdisciplinary style of teaching to train all specialists in medicine, including nursing and allied health
personnel, concerning the special needs of the elderly
patient. Such a faculty should provide information, teach
skills, and influence positive attitudes toward care of the
elderly. Continuing education for all health professionals
and educating the public are included in the responsibilities
of the geriatric faculty.

Should our academic medical center develop a geriatric
inpatient unit? It is beneficial to program development to
concentrate selected elderly patients in a common setting
in order to do effective teaching and research, rather than
to disperse patients throughout the hospital. Elderly
patients benefit as the environment is attuned to their
varied medical, social, and psychological problems. This
same grouping of patients may not be desirable in a community hospital without a geriatrics program. Careful,
ongoing evaluation of the geriatric inpatient setting is
essential to ensure that patients and unit are not
promoting a sense of isolation or an unfavorable stereotype.

The tertiary care nature of the academic medical center
tends to preclude the student from gaining experience in
long-term care of patients with chronic illness. The
geriatrics teaching program offers the student an opportunity
to study all ramifications of chronic illness and should
include experience in the geriatric inpatient unit, nursing
home, ambulatory care setting, and patient's home. The
student will come to understand psychological, social, and
economic problems as well as appreciate individual patient
adaptations to chronic illness.

What research programs should be pursued when problems of the aged are considered? The search for values for normal body function is critical in different age groups. Therefore, biological changes that occur with normal aging process need to be elucidated. Research in the health services area should include measurements or evaluations of appropriate settings in which health care can be delivered in the most efficient and satisfactory manner. Are there better means to fund health services for aged? Understanding of pathological changes that occur in and affect the organs require development of individual research programs in chronic diseases that threaten the elderly. Psychological changes that occur in the elderly need careful review. Since the elderly spend millions of dollars per year on varieties of vitamins and patent medicines, are these of value, or are we wasting the elderly person's retirement income? The federal government has organized an agency to assist academic medical centers pursue research programs. The National Institute on Aging, established by Congress in 1974, will lead the way and establish necessary evaluation teams to consider merits and funding of various research programs.

Academic medical centers will be in the forefront in developing educational, research, and model health care programs for the aged. An example is the volume at hand, the result of two conferences on aging conducted jointly by the University of Virginia and the Veterans Administration Medical Center in Salem, Virginia. Papers from these conferences will be distributed to a variety of health care providers and institutions in order to provide latest medical advances and relevant information concerning caring for the aged. Information gathered at these conferences will find its way into newspapers, thereby presenting to the general public the concerns of the medical profession regarding the elderly and the accomplishments made in this area.

The University of Virginia Medical School and the Veterans Administration Medical Center have been partners for many years in developing and carrying out important health care programs in hopes that the health and welfare of citizens of Virginia and the nation would be improved. It is to this end that these conferences and the publication of their papers are dedicated.

Norman J. Knorr, M.D.
Charlottesville, VA 22908

Preface

This book is written for people who care for the elderly:
physicians, nurses, social workers, dietitians, hospital
and nursing home administrators, agencies on aging, health
planners, and families. It combines comprehensive, "hands-
on," care of the elderly and their underlying demographic,
socioeconomic, and medical circumstances.

The concept of this book has changed several times.
The Salem Veterans Administration Medical Center and the
University of Virginia School of Medicine jointly presented
a conference entitled "Aging and Health" in September 1978.
We were assigned the role of preparing a "proceedings."
The conference had two different formats: plenary papers
and discussion groups on various problems of the elderly.
A choice had to be made. We could have quickly published
a "proceedings" composed only of the papers. Review of the
conference material, however, showed that we would lose the
opportunity of including the panel presentations based on
the rich experience of our participants. We chose the
slower, more difficult route of including the panel discussions. This required months of transcribing tapes and
more months of integrating the messages. When our second
"Aging and Health" conference came in 1979, we added four
more papers from that meeting. Later we added one previously published paper because it fit so well with others
on home health care. We now feel we are presenting a
multidisciplinary, multiauthored handbook on care.

A number of themes thread the book. The most pervasive
is the intermingling of social and medical aspects of well-
being with the quality of living. Since the elderly are
the consumers of our care, we felt it important to include
the insights of a number of superb providers who are themselves elderly. The need for providers from many disciplines to integrate and focus on individual patients is
emphasized. There is a gap between what is known and what
can be delivered in the care of the elderly. Some state and
regional approaches have been presented, using Virginia as
a model.

Harold B. Haley, M.D.
Patricia A. Keenan
Roanoke, Virginia 24014

Acknowledgments

This book is the result of the effort of many people. The concept of our jointly sponsored conferences and this publication began with Dr. Francis L. Brochu and Dr. William D. Poe. Dr. Brochu has been the prime organizer and director of our conferences. Dr. Poe's long experience and foundation thinking in geriatrics underlie much of our planning. Dr. E. Gifford Ammermann helped in the editing. Other active contributors on our committee include, from the Salem Veterans Administration Medical Center, Dr. William E. Reefe, Chief, Medical Service; Dr. Nina Magier, Psychiatrist; Arnold Simmons, Chief, Social Work Service; and Ms. Anna Lee Chalfante, Chief Nurse. From the University of Virginia, Dr. Richard H. Lindsay, Director, Division of Geriatric Medicine, and Dr. Oscar Thorup, Associate Dean for Continuing Medical Education. And Mr. Frank H. Mays, Executive Director, Southwest Virginia Health Systems Agency.

Mr. Hugh Davis, Director of the Salem Veterans Administration Medical Center, and Dr. Norman J. Knorr, Dean, University of Virginia School of Medicine, have been supportive and participated in the development of new geriatric programs in their institutions. Dr. Knorr has particularly supported this publication.

We wish to thank our authors for their thoughts and cooperation. Special mention should be made of Dr. Ralph Goldman, Chief of Extended Care, Veterans Administration Central Office. His three scholarly contributions add depth.

The American Geriatric Society and the League of Older Americans cosponsored our conferences. We cherish their collaboration.

The two conferences went well. Mr. Robert Pafford and his staff provided outstanding audiovisual service. Mr. Ted Smith handled well the details of the meeting. Operations were carried out by a dedicated staff composed of Emma Caldwell, Lorena Garnand, and Helena Kerfoot of the Veterans Administration Medical Center in Salem, Virginia, and Mary Lou Currier from the University of Virginia School of Medicine in Charlottesville.

It is impossible to list all who helped, but we would like to thank our typists, Ruth P. Scott, Mondia E. Dyer, and Suzanne Craig, who often acted as eagle-eyed proofreaders.

Among librarians, Lucy Glenn of the Roanoke Memorial Hospitals library, Jean Kennedy and Mary Ann Tatman of the Veterans Administration Medical Center Library, and Lenore Schnaitman of the University of Virginia Health Sciences Library verified references and guided us in our research.

Part I

The Health and Social Status of Elderly Persons

INTRODUCTION

Harold B. Haley

Perry Kendig correlates the status of elderly people, both as individuals and as groups. Dr. Kendig gives a sensitive discussion of the concerns of a physically and mentally healthy retiree. What are the problems? What are the compensations and rewards? What kinds of adjustments have to be made?

Maggie Kuhn, an articulate spokeswoman, narrates viewpoints of the elderly as a group, outlining their problems, pluses, and solutions.

Nina Magier details the myths that have grown in our culture concerning the elderly.

The environmental and cultural problems of the elderly from a societal standpoint are recounted by Nancy Lohmann.

Ralph Goldman, in the first of three papers, relates specific geriatric health problems to the social environment and explores risk factors and dying in detail.

Drs. Maddox and Steel explore these problems and search for solutions. George Maddox relates three ongoing revolutions and outlines what is necessary to solve these interrelated, social and health problems.

Knight Steel shows that in solving some aspects of the health problems of the elderly, the M.D. serves as gatekeeper.

CHAPTER 1

RUMINATIONS OF A RETIREE

OR

LESSONS IN TAKING THE BITTER WITH THE BETTER

Perry Fridy Kendig

My qualifications for this paper are scanty. Although some
of my best friends are physicians, I know little about medicine. I have never really worked with the aging other than
with relatives and a few close friends. However, I do have
one ineluctable advantage: I am retired, and have been for
about four years. I can't be accused of a purely theoretical
approach. I've been there!

I feel a gentle undercurrent of uneasiness about this
paper that I can explain by citing an old and shopworn joke.
Abe Lincoln asked a fellow townsman, who had been tarred and
feathered and ridden out of town on a rail, what his reactions were. The chap replied: "Well, if it wasn't for the
honor of the thing, I'd just have soon walked."

The full title of this paper resembles the titles of
the early novels in English and American literature in that
it has a subtitle. Samuel Richardson's novel in 1740, often
considered the first real novel written in English, is
entitled Pamela, or Virtue Rewarded. Roanoke College
Library's rarest book, a romantic fiction by Judge Jesse
Lynch Holman published in 1810, is entitled The Prisoners
of Niagara, or Errors of Education. The full title of this
paper is "Ruminations of a Retiree, or Lessons in Taking
the Bitter with the Better."

Since I hope to end this paper on a positive note, I
shall discuss "the bitter" first, leaving "the better" for
the end.

First, we will consider some less desirable aspects
of retirement. Dumb questions asked in kindness and with
a real desire to be pleasant and interested. Americans use
questions as a kind of greeting ritual, for example, "Hi,
how are you?" This is a greeting, not a genuine question
(unless you are recently released from a hospital). The
answer to this is general and is usually, "Fine."

If you don't believe this is a greeting rather than
a question, just start to tell the next busy person who
greets you thus how you really are, and in detail. In
less than a minute his eyes will begin to glaze and he
will glance at his watch.

This is why many old people seem boring to the young.
Just ask some old lady how she feels some day and lean back,
because you asked for it and you're going to get it. She'll
tell you!

Another of these greeting questions that I react poorly to is: "Wha da ya know?" The expected answer is: "Not much, how about you?" But professors often don't get off so easily because their greeters usually add: "With all that education, you ought to know something!" I worked out an answer for that one; I simply say: "Chaucer died in 1400." If I were in your shoes, I believe I'd say: "Aspirin is a useful drug."

After retirement these greeting questions continue, but two new ones are added: "What are you doing with yourself these days?" I have discovered no short answer for this one yet, but I'm working on it.

A second more intense version often used by harassed overachievers and workaholics is: "How in the word do you keep busy?" with a very heavy emphasis on the word 'busy'. I've got an answer for this one. I simply say, "I don't!" A true workaholic then looks at me stricken, as though I have just given him a hard rabbit punch on his left kidney. So much for questions.

The waning of one's powers is another less desirable aspect of retirement. There is a physical deterioration which seems to happen to different people and different sexes at different times and at different paces. There is a waning of sexual power and potency—and then even desire—and finally even interest in the subject. This varies greatly among individuals; but if one lives long enough, one will almost certainly experience some stage of it. This can be embarrassing at best and downright humiliating at worst. (I refuse to discuss those yogurt-eating 90-year-old south Russians with 26-year-old wives and stairstep children ranging from one to 70 years of age. In the pictures many of those young wives have a very foxy look around the eyes. Yes, I'm a male chauvinist, and have a necktie to prove it.)

The waning of physical strength is serious for a farmer, not too significant for a professor. The waning of nimbleness, agility. This one bothers me. I am older. I am more arthritic. I cannot dance nearly as well as I used to, and I haven't been on a horse for years, although I still watch horse shows from the rail with wet and envious eyes. The waning of sense perceptions: sight, hearing, taste, smell, and touch. All become in time second or third rate. This diminishes one's enjoyment of many fine things.

The waning of one's mental powers and emotional balance and stability (I am not referring to out-and-out senility, which I observe to be often a euphoric state, but to the twilight zone between full powers and full senility). Memory fails. Proper names go first. Maybe tomorrow I'll find out why. The desire to listen weakens. Retired people tend to talk too much in general and to reminisce too much in particular. (One of the nicest things you can do

for a retired person is to listen to him--or her--and listen
attentively and sympathetically. It's hard, but do it.)
     The financial bind is another less desirable aspect of
retirement. This one gets a lot of publicity, especially
in these times of serious inflation. I confess that I am
uneasy about stagflation. In times of recession, prices
should go down; in the big depression of my youth, prices
went very low. When I was in graduate school in Philadelphia
in the early 1930s, my food budget was $1.00 per day--and
that was eating in cafeterias and restaurants. It called for
25¢ for breakfast, 25¢ for lunch and 50¢ for dinner. If you
went to a tea room for dinner, it ran 55¢ to $1.00 with a
10% tip for the waitress. Old folks on pensions and fixed
incomes got along fine in 1934, thank you. It doesn't seem
to work that way any more. Breakfasts in Roanoke run from
about $1.50 to $5.00.
     I believe that in this great, rich country of ours,
thousands of retired folks are going to be cold or hungry
or both this winter and I don't like that one little bit.
What can these folks do? Get a job. OK, fine. What sort
of job? Bag boy in the supermarket? If single, marry a
rich mate? A tough way to make a living! Be a consultant?
(I'm a consultant, but no one ever consults me except to ask
what sort of strange bird is eating their expensive sun-
flower seed. It seems inappropriate to send them a bill for
that service, doesn't it?) Go on welfare of one form or
other? Start to use capital? When it's gone, throw yourself on the mercy of the welfare state or turn on the gas.
Not very appealing prospects.
     Retired people have much more time for eschatological
thinking. And this doesn't cheer them up much either, for
the eschaton is a lot closer for us than it is for most of
you.
     Well, before I dissolve into tears, let us look at
things retired persons seem to miss most. Generous income
is missed, which we mentioned. Perquisites, I use the
clergy word here, are missed. This is not my opinion alone;
I have discussed this with some of my trustees who retired
near to the time I did. This is what we agreed we missed.
A good private secretary, an expense account, and staff
who will take care of routine while you think about what
must be done for the future so that your organization will
be better in the next decade. If you were successful in
your job, you felt a sense of satisfaction and importance
that it is difficult as a retired person to earn or enjoy.
In other words, before you retire you are somebody and you
know who you are. One man put it this way: "You have something to get up for and you believe that 'something' is a
matter of some importance. It's difficult for most retired
folks to hang on to these sorts of perquisites and, frankly,
most of us miss them."

Friends, there is a brighter side. Let's look at "the better" as we conclude our little essay on life in retirement. I am going to be personal and subjective here because I can only recount what has seemed most different and pleasurable to me. Freedom from reponsibility is a "better" part of retirement. I understand that I am still responsible for myself, and, to some extent, for my family. But I am no longer responsible to an outside organization that can court-martial or discharge me at will.

There are several factors in this freedom that I have particularly enjoyed. I am no longer "on duty" 24 hours a day, day after day, year after year. Horrible examples abound. With one exception, I have not had to ask my friends for money for four whole years. They no longer have to grab their pocketbooks when they see me enter the club. I like that. I am free NOT to serve as president of ANYTHING ever again. God be praised! I enjoy my freedom from rigid scheduling. No longer do I have to attend evening meetings called by someone else. (Fortunately, my physician backs me up in this. And, at monthly bill paying time, his name leads all the rest.) My sleeping habits have become like those of an old retired bird dog. I can get up when I want to, go to bed when I want to, and take a nap whenever I feel the need. I get between 6 and 8 hours sleep out of 24 on my own schedule. I like this freedom, and I don't think I abuse it much.

I enjoy having more time to devote to my life-long hobby: ornithology. My mother was good at birding and I caught the fever from her. It was the first merit badge I earned in scouting. I have studied ornithology for credit at my alma mater and taught it as a noncredit course at Roanoke College. I like birds, I like the outdoors (I'm a country boy), but most of all I like my fellow birders, a gentle and genial lot.

I enjoy having more time to think--to think long thoughts that have nothing to do with decision making, the plight of private higher education, or problem solving.

Professor James Harvey Robinson many years ago identified four kinds of thinking. I can now afford to spend a little less time on decision making and rationalization and more time in reverie and even occasionally in creative thinking. I enjoy this.

Well, my friends, these are the ruminations on retirement by a retiree that were promised you. I hope I did not bore you younger folks. I won't apologize for being personal and subjective, because that's the only way I could handle it.

CHAPTER 2

MYTHS PERTAINING TO AGING

Nina G. Magier

False beliefs and prejudices die slowly; when alive, they
contribute to the development of negative attitudes. These
attitudes influence our relationships with people and contribute to the development of feelings about ourselves.

By the end of this century we will have over 30 million
elderly, 10% of the population of the United States. We are
a youth-oriented society. The elderly are considered physically disabled and mentally impaired, if not completely
incompetent, and are looked down upon.

This attitude is not only reflected in difficulty obtaining a job after age 40 or getting insurance coverage,
but in our language. The word "senescence" (for normal
phase of life) is rarely used in professional literature.
Instead, the word "senile" is popular in colloquial language,
carrying the connotation "What can you expect of him or her?"
Common derogatory expressions reflecting the same devastating
attitude are "foggy," "crutch," "witch," etc., with the addition of adjectives like "dirty old man" or "out of her head"
if the elderly person happens to demonstrate an interest in
the opposite sex.

As an example, I was asked to see a 58-year-old man in
a psychiatric consultation because "He is getting senile."
He pinched a female employee--a kind of behavior that produces
a glow if a younger man does the same. One is admired for
virility; another is considered senile and ought to have tranquilizers. This is one example of numerous myths that will
be presented.

Myth no. 1: The elderly are supposed to be asexual.
Nothing can be farther from the truth. One need not go to
Florida for verification. Some elderly, particularly women,
state they are enjoying sex more than ever before because
they are free from family responsibilities, a busy and hectic
life, fear of pregnancy, and they can relax.

Myth no. 2: The elderly are demented (dementare--
deprive of mind). Growing old is equated with losing one's
mental faculties: ability to think, understand, reason,
reflect, have will, judgment, perceive, recognize, ability
to acquire ideas, recollect, remember, and comprehend. All
of these are covered in the word "cognition," from
cognoscere--to know. Younger persons are not always logical
and are forgetful, too. But, if an elderly person forgets,
not only do others remark but the persons says, "I am getting
senile." So deeply is this myth ingrained that it could be
a self-fulfilling prophecy. This is an anxiety-producing
feeling because impairment of mental functions or losing

one's mind means ceasing to exist as a rational individual
being. The famous French philosopher Descartes summed it up
in a short sentence: Cogito ergo sum--"I think, hence I
exist."

In reality, aging does not bring mental deterioration.
In a research testing situation, 45 professors (age 60 to
80) were compared with 45 younger colleagues on the faculty
(age 25 to 35). The elderly group did much better on vocab-
ulary and general knowledge. Throughout history many people
have made outstanding contributions to mankind at a later
age: Sophocles; Galileo; Cervantes; Harvey; Thomas Jefferson;
Benjamin Franklin (who at age 78 invented bifocals when he
got tired of wearing two pairs of glasses--one for far sight
and the other for near sight--and changing them constantly);
Voltaire; Goethe; Tolstoy; Verdi (who composed Falstaff at
age 82); Churchill; Adenauer (at age 85 pulled Germany out
of ashes and brought reconciliation with France); and Grandma
Moses, who became famous at the sunset of her life. At age
78 she gave up embroidery because of arthritis and she tried
the brush and a one-woman art exhibit followed. Grandma Moses
kept painting until her death at age 101. Rubenstein, at
age 90, kept captivating audiences with piano concerts flaw-
lessly performed. There are many more remarkable elderly.
My most unforgettable vacation was with my father, age 92.
It was like taking a postgraduate course in literature and
history, including contemporary. President Franklin Roose-
velt paid his respects to Justice Holmes on his 92d birthday. He found him reading Plato and was so amazed that he
exclaimed, "Why do you read Plato, Mr. Justice?" A simple,
yet profound, reply came, "To exercise my mind, Mr. President." Yes, indeed, if athletes exercise their muscles in
order to maintain and strengthen performance, we all need to
exercise our minds in order to maintain our thinking
capacities.

Myth no. 3: "You cannot teach an old dog new tricks."
This statement is erroneous. Hundreds of elderly are going
to school now, learning successfully, enriching their lives,
and going into new enterprises. Also, there are tricks
that only the "old dogs" know how to perform.

Myth no. 4: The old are rigid, not flexible. This is
false. My experience and that of others has shown that the
elderly adapt themselves to different losses, circumstances,
and continuous changes. Yes, the elderly are flexible and
adaptable.

Myth no. 5: The belief that people who were spared
blows of fate grow old more successfully is also not correct.
In fact, they are more vulnerable. Exposure to stress calls
for coping and learning how to cope, and provides an opportunity for growth and development of stamina. From the
moment we take our first breath, we face changes. They continue throughout life and do not end at age 65 with retirement.

Challenges continue and the majority of the elderly are meeting them admirably.

Myth no. 6: This refers to "arteriosclerotic brains"--another derogatory remark because the aging process includes arteriosclerotic changes. Whenever intellectual impairment happens, it is not always due to arteriosclerosis. Now we know that only approximately 7% of those that develop difficulties are due to arteriosclerosis. The rest are due to multiple or various causes and 37% are treatable and reversible (important awareness for all of us).

Myth no. 7: The elderly are not treatable or, worse yet, why treat them--they are going to die soon, anyhow? Death comes to all but at different times. Who is to say when one is going to die? Now we know that what is treatable in the young can be treated in the elderly, and what is treatable is preventable. The elderly respond well to treatment, not only physically but emotionally, if given attention, a chance, and hope.

Myth no. 8: The elderly are "hypochondriacs." This is a more subtle issue. Some young people are, too! Depression may be in disguise. What frequently happens is that the elderly are falsely perceived as hypochondriacs and dismissed with, "There is nothing wrong with you," while, in reality, he or she is misunderstood. A physical complaint could be a form of communication, a matter of expressing the need for attention--the need to have someone to turn to, to be heard, be trusted, not criticized or laughted at.

Myth no. 9: Mental illness in the elderly is irreversible. The attitude, "Put him or her away," or declare incompetent, is not only false but catastrophic. Mental illnesses in the aged are treatable, could be reversible (completely or partially), or can be arrested with dramatic improvement in functioning and quality of life. Special consideration and knowledge are needed but attitude is most important. This is a challenge.

Myth no. 10: The elderly are a risk at work. The record shows that the elderly have fewer accidents, are more loyal, less wasteful, and show less absenteeism than the young.

Myth no. 11: The elderly are unable to grow; they live in the past. This is not true. The body is aging but not the interest in life.

Myth no. 12: The aged are in their second childhood. This overlooks the fact that changes in behavior could be symptomatic of some developing illness. Symptomatic mental illness is now well recognized due to infection, malnutrition, electrolyte imbalance, medication--whatever. It may be the first symptom of failing heart function or endocrine disorder. In the child everybody looks for a cause, but the elderly are called childish, dismissed as senile, and are doomed.

How can one survive without hope? Negative attitudes
that play a considerable role in the development of chronic
psychological disabilities in the aged have to be changed.
If there is a tomorrow for the young, there is a tomorrow
for the aging.

The elusive Fountain of Youth has not been found. But,
with the dispelling of harmful myths and better knowledge,
understanding, and constructive attitudes, we can improve
the quality of life of the elderly. Sunset can be as beautiful as sunrise!

CHAPTER 3

THE PATIENT TALKS BACK

Margaret E. Kuhn

There is a great deal that we "Gray Panthers," radical, wrinkled, old folks and young folks, have to say and to do with you who are part of the medical establishment. My credentials are having arthritis in both hands and in both knees, living through two bouts of cancer, being seventy-three years old, traveling about a hundred thousand miles a year, and, finally, last month completing my second visit to the People's Republic of China.

This interdisciplinary conference symbolizes a profound change that has occurred in our society and illustrates we can communicate with each other from different vantage points and discover our true humanity in the process. You might title this paper, "The Way It Looks from between the Sheets." It is a different view of life and of the medical establishment from between the sheets. And, if any of you haven't had that opportunity lately, I would recommend it for a brief interval. Aging is the one thing that all of us share. It is the one thing that gives us a broad-scale perspective on the whole condition of life. Aging begins at the moment of life, aging begins at the moment of birth and ends with rigor mortis. Whatever time boundaries you put upon it, aging is the universal experience that all living things share.

I learned that dinosaurs had arthritis. This has helped me deal with my own wrinkled fingers and gnarled hands. Those disabling and persistent human conditions challenge those of us who are between the sheets and those of you who stand outside the sheets.

Maybe, together, we can do some extraordinary things to systems, to change ourselves and to change society as a whole. All of you are getting old. My friends in social gerontology, in trying to be completely pure and objective, have disassociated themselves from their own humanity and have looked at us as aging guinea pigs, instead of realizing that we are all aging together. The aging process includes all of us, not only human animals, but all other animals. Aging puts us in touch with the plants, with everything that grows, there is this human dimension of aging. Recycling, redeeming, reclaiming--old houses, old towns, old people-- is part of the newness of this age. All around me are radical critiques of the extraordinary waste that we have had in our society for too long. Although recycling paper, metal, and water now, we still throw human beings away when they are old and sick and somehow nonproductive. We are involved in an important salvaging, recycling operation that could have an impact upon society. What are you doing in the course of your daily work? You who are social workers,

nurses, researchers, physicians, administrators, and thera-
pists, involved in the delicate and important part of
rehabilitation, directed to the old warriors. Are you bringing an extra dimension of human compassion and concern?

Rereading C. Wright Mills's Sociological Imagination
after thirty years reinforced my fondness for his ideals.
Mills was a distinguished sociologist at Columbia University
who wrote some things that bear upon this process of recycling,
redeeming, reclaiming, making new and whole what is fractured
and broken and sick. Mills states that each of us has our
own biography. We live our lives, and many of us live our
lives in a very private way. Our own careers, our own
families, our own professional advancement, the dynamics of
the rather confined human situation in which we live are
private. That is our biography. Each of us is a part of
history. History and biography intersect in you and me and
in the events that we are a part of and that we ourselves
create. There are no really personal, private problems or
troubles without a societal resolution and solution and
approach. He also reminds us that there is no global issue,
like war, nuclear destruction, unemployment, or galloping
inflation that can be fully comprehended in its broad societal, economic, political aspects without realizing what
these global issues do to people. The smallest, the meek-
est, and the most frail of us are all a part of human history, world history. You and I find our biographies inter-
secting with history and our own histories being seen in a
new light because of this intersection.

Oral history interests me. Some fascinating oral history has been written, spoken, and recorded here in
the Blue Ridge Mountains. You who are in daily contact with
old people who have been a part of tragic and exciting and
exhilarating events have access to their interesting oral
history. A part of the therapy and rehabilitation program
could include some oral histories recorded on tape, brought
out from forgotten memories of people you work with, that
could illuminate their past and inform the present, and point
to what we ought to be doing in the future.

When I can't sleep at night, science fiction books
offer peace. A favorite, Colin Wilson's The Philosopher's
Stone is exciting science fiction that identifies the secret,
the key to long life, the key to longevity as "value experience" (V.E.). Wilson thinks "V.E.'s" are more important to
survival and good health in old age than "I.Q.'s." Each of
us has them, but we only get hold of them when we have looked
at our own roots and valued our past. You who are dealing
with large blocks of history, in many instances tragic
history, that the people you work with have been a part of,
have access to unlocking the secret of a good age. Hopefully, this interposition of history and biography, the value
of experience, can be seen in a new light.

You, as a group with influence, power, access to enor-
mous amounts of research money, and many acres of medical
facilities, have a corner on more living history than any
other group. Have you thought about that? You see the
results of war related injuries and related sickness, and,
most of all, the experiences of terrifying wars. You have,
within the capacity of your own institutions, the most powerful lobby for peace that the world has ever known. If there
is to be more human history ahead, there has to be a lobby
of peace seekers and peace makers based on experiences of
those who have known firsthand the horrors of war. To save
our planet and to save the human race.

References

(1)   Mills, C. Wright. Sociological Imagination. New York:
       Oxford University Press, 1967.
(2)   Wilson, Colin. The Philosopher's Stone. New York:
       Warner Books, 1974.

CHAPTER 4

AGING AND SOCIAL PROBLEMS

Nancy L. Lohmann

A basic assumption in gerontology is that the nature of the
problems encountered when working with older people requires
a multi- and inter-disciplinary approach. No one discipline
encompasses all the knowledge that is needed, if we are to
assist older people successfully. The professional social
worker's role is to identify some of the social problems
experienced by the aged that influence their health status
and health care. Income status and social relationships
and satisfactions of aged will be discussed emphasizing
status of rural and small town aged.

Income

The income status of the aged has been of concern to social
gerontologists. It was economic deprivation of the elderly
that resulted in creation of the social insurance program
called Social Security and in creation of social welfare
programs such as Supplemental Security Income (SSI). Income
status of the aged affects development of disease and illness in older people by limiting their diet and access to
preventive and therapeutic health care.
     In spite of long-standing income programs, older people
are still relatively economically deprived. Brotman
provides us with median income data for 1975:

	Median income for families	Median income for individuals
Over 65 years	$ 8,057	$3,311
Under 65 years	$14,698	$6,460

When comparing income of the elderly to poverty lines
established by the federal government, we find that while the
elderly are approximately 10% of the population, they consti-
tute 13% of those who are poor. Of the total aged population,
15.3% are below poverty line and another 25% are "near poor,"
or very close to that line (1).
     There are subpopulations of the aged who are among the
poor and "near poor." The minority aged, unrelated individuals (who tend to be older women), and rural aged are more
likely to be poor. Among rural aged, rural nonfarm aged tend
to be more disadvantaged then rural farm or urban aged
     The impact of income on prevention of illness and
disease is multifold. First, an inadequate income often

results in an inadequate diet. Inadequacy of the diet, in
turn, results in a physical condition that leads the aged to
be more susceptible to disease. Secondly, an inadequate income often prevents the aged from receiving preventive medical care. If choice is between shelter and a medical check-
up, most older people will choose shelter. This lack of
coverage for preventive health care by health insurance
programs, such as Medicare, is a further deterrent to receiving such care.

Income also affects health care received when illness
or disease are present. It was hoped that Medicare and
Medicaid would result in improved access to health care by
older people. However, these programs have fallen short of
our expectations. For example, in 1970 only 43% of total
health bill for the aged was paid for by Medicare (3).
Magnusen and Segal have indicated that "in fact, inflation
has been so rapid that the elderly are now paying more dollars
out of their own pockets for health care than they did before
Medicare was adopted in 1965! According to a 1973 Social
Security Administration report, the average elderly person's
out-of-pocket health costs have increased from $234 to $276
in six years (1966-1972)" (4).

Often, out-of-pocket health costs paid by older people
are more than we, with our relatively adequate incomes, pay
under health insurance programs that cover us.

Social Relationships

Another problem that has an effect on health status is social
relationships. Discussions of such relationships often
emphasize their absence through use of the term "social isolation." However, an examination of research findings on
such relationships suggest that opportunity for social contact may be present to a larger degree than is often realized.

Studies of family relationships of older people have
found that about 83% of the aged have at least one child
within an hour's distance. In addition to physical proximity
of a child, about 80% see a child once a week or more (5).
Thus, most older people do have both physical access to, and
actual contact with, an adult child. This relationships may
serve to reduce social isolation of the older person. Little
research has been done on the meaning of such contact, so we
do not know if it actually does reduce feelings of isolation.

There are some rural-urban differences in such contacts.
Rural older people are less likely to have children living
in the same community and visit their children less frequently than do their urban counterparts (6-7). ("Rural"
refers to an area of 2,500 inhabitants or less.)

Strong community ties represent a form of compensation
for rural aged, given their greater relative isolation from
their children. Rural older people are more likely to engage
in informal visiting, to know a large number of people within

their community, to have a large number of friends and to be satisfied with their community than are urban aged (8). These relationships with friends may reduce feelings of social isolation. Conversely, urban aged are less likely to engage in informal visiting or have many friends. Studies of friendship among urban aged indicate that 40% visit friends once a week or more often (9). Most studies have indicated the wish of urban aged for more friends and more of the types of social interaction that takes place among friends (10-11).

With regard to one form of social relationship, the marital relationship, older women are especially disadvantaged. Among those over 65 years of age, 79% of men are married but only about 39% of women are married (12). For most older men, the social relationship of marriage and other relationships that often accompany it, contact with other couples, etc., are still intact. For most older women, however, the social relationship of marriage and the accompanying relationships are not. While social relationships other than the marital one may partially compensate for the loss of a partner, they will not replace a duadic relationship. Relationships with children, siblings, neighbors, and other friends cannot fill the isolation brought about by loss of one's husband. Evidence of failure of these relationships to compensate can be found in lowered morale which persists for up to ten years after loss of a spouse among widows.

The quality of social aspects of life, including the quality of social relationships, is often measured through use of such constructs as life satisfaction, adjustment, and morale. Efforts to identify factors which influence life satisfaction of the aged have been a central focus of gerontological research and theorizing for the past thirty years (13). One factor that has been extensively examined is that of health status. Eleven studies that have found a positive relationship between health and life satisfaction have been identified (14-25). In several instances, when multivariate techniques such as path analysis or multiple regression were used to identify variance in life satisfaction, health was found to be one primary factor (16, 17, 24). However, relationship between health and satisfaction may not be as clearcut as is assumed.

Data which suggest that health produces life satisfaction is either correlational in nature or is the result of efforts to statistically explain variance. It is often presumed that correlational data represent one form of evidence that health produces given levels of life satisfaction. However, since these data are merely correlational and thus do not meet all requirements for causal proof (26), the direction of the relationship is a common-sense assumption. One could as easily assume the direction is the other way: that levels of life satisfaction produce given levels of

health. When we go beyond correlating these two factors
and attempt to statistically explain variance or direction,
we are also imposing our assumptions about direction of relationship on the data. Here, too, it could be that direction
is the opposite of the way we have assumed. Rather than a
high level of health producing a high level of life satisfaction, it is a high level of life satisfaction that produces
a high level of health.

The theoretical possibility that relationship may run
opposite the direction, that is often assumed, suggests the
importance for health professionals to be as aware of a
patient's social and life-satisfaction status as they are of
their health status. For example, it may be that a patient's
health status can be better changed by changing the social
relationships than by introducing some new form of medical
treatment. The possible bidirectional relationship between
health and life satisfaction is one that cannot be ignored.

In conclusion, it must be reemphasized that the multidisciplinary nature of gerontology and of caring for the
aged means that contributions of all disciplines must be
taken into account. Social disciplines could identify some
social problems which negatively affect the aged and their
health status. Two such problems have been identified today:
impact of income on health status and access to health care
and impact of social relationships on health care. As health
professionals care for the aged, they need to bear in mind
the multidirectional relationship that may exist between
these factors and health.

References

(1) Brotman, H. B. "Income and Poverty in the Older Popu-
     lation in 1975." Gerontologist 17:23-26, 1977.
(2) Atchley, R. C. Rural Environments and Aging. Washing-
     ton, D.C.: Gerontological Society, 1975, pp. 1-9.
(3) Cooper, B. C., and M. F. McGee. "Medical Care Outlays
     for Three Age Groups: Young, Intermediate and Aged."
     Social Security Bulletin, 12, 1971.
(4) Magnusen, W., and E. Segal. How Much for Health?
     Washington, D.C.: Robert B. Luce, 1974, p. 23.
(5) Stehouwer, J. "Relations between Generations and the
     Three-Generation Household in Denmark." In Social
     Structure and Family: Generational Relations, edited
     by Ethel Shanas and Gordon Streib. Englewood Cliffs,
     N.J.: Prentice-Hall, 1965, pp. 142-62.
(6) Bultena, G. "Rural-Urban Differences in the Familial
     Interaction of the Aged." Rural Sociology 34:5-15, 1969.
(7) Youmans, G. "Aging Patterns in a Rural and an Urban
     Area of Kentucky." Bulletin 681, Lexington, Ky.: U.S.
     Department of Agriculture. Agricultural Experiment
     Station, 1963.

(8) Powers, E. A., P. Keith, and W. Goudy. "Family Relationships and Friendships." In Rural Environments and Aging, edited by R. C. Atchley. Washington, D.C.: Gerontological Society, 1975, pp. 67-90.

(9) Shanas, E. The Health of Older People: A Social Survey. Cambridge, Mass.: Harvard University Press, 1962.

(10) Hunter, W. W. and H. Maurice. Older People Tell Their Story. Ann Arbor: Institute for Human Adjustment, 1953.

(11) Rosow, I. Social Integration of the Aged. New York: Free Press, 1967.

(12) Facts about Older Americans. Publication No. (OHD) 78-20006, Washington, D.C.: U.S. Department of Health, Education and Welfare, 1977.

(13) Lohmann, N. Comparison of Life Satisfaction, Morale and Adjustment Scales on an Elderly Population. Diss., Brandeis University, Waltham, Mass., 1975.

(14) Britton, J. O., and J. H. Britton. "Factors Related to the Adjustment of Retired YMCA Secretaries." Journal of Gerontology 6:34-38, 1951.

(15) Cavan, R. S., and E. W. Burgess. Personal Adjustment in Old Age. Chicago: Science Research Associates, 1949.

(16) Edwards, J. N., and D. L. Klemmack. "Correlates of Life Satisfaction: A Re-examination." Journal of Gerontology 28:499-502, 1973.

(17) Falkman, P. W. "Objective, Subjective and Continuity Correlates of Life Satisfaction in an Elderly Population." Dissertation Abstracts International 33:8A: 4556-4557, 1973.

(18) Havinghurst, R. J., and R. Albrecht. Older People, New York: Longmans, Green Co., 1953.

(19) Maddox, G. "Activity and Morale: A Longitudinal Study of Selected Elderly Subjects." Social Forces 42:195-204, 1963.

(20) Maddox, G., and C. Eisdorfer. "Some Correlates of Activity and Morale among the Elderly." Social Forces 40:254-260, 1962.

(21) Messer, M. "Race Differences in Selected Attitudinal Dimensions of the Elderly." Gerontologist 8:245-49, 1968.

(22) Seymour, G. O. "Activity Level, the Sense of Personal Autonomy and Life Satisfaction in Old Age." Dissertation Abstracts International 33:5B: 2331-2332, 1973.

(23) Streib, G. "Morale of the Retired." Social Problems 3:270-276, 1956.

(24) Thompson, G. B. "Work versus Leisure Roles: An Investigation of Morale among Employed and Retired Men." Journal of Gerontology 28:339-344, 1973.

(25) Zibbell, R. A. "Activity Level, Future Time Perspective and Life Satisfaction in Old Age." Dissertation Abstracts International 32:7B; 4198-4199, 1972.

(26) Blalock, H. M., Jr., Causal Inferences in Nonexperimental Research. Chapel Hill: University of North Carolina Press, 1964.

CHAPTER 5

THE AGING PROCESS AND THE GERONTOLOGIST

Ralph Goldman

What is a gerontologist? A geron, or gerontos, is an
old man. An iatros is a physician. So a "geriatrician"
is a physician for old men. Another word, iatria, means
treatment, so geriatrics could also be interpreted as treatment of old men. On the other hand, gerontology derives from
the word gerontos and the word logos, which means dis-
course upon or, by implication, the study of aging. As
geriatrics is the care of aged, gerontology is the study of
aging process. While geriatrics can use the products of
gerontology in studying the aging process, it is necessary
to start earlier than at the time of old age in order to
know from whence changes have come. We have some other
important definitions. One is the concept of life span.
Life span is not how long we live; life span is the longest
survival of an individual of its species. We are much more
interested in life expectation, that is, average duration
of life of individuals in a given cohort, or population.
       Life is a sequence of gains and losses, incremental
and decremental changes. Growth and development are associated with a predominance of gains over losses, but, unfortunately, from adulthood on, losses exceed gains. At first,
this is at a slow rate that accelerates with increasing age.
The current concept of gerontologists seems to point to the
direction of a built-in biologic clock that limits ultimate
survival. We will now examine some of the overt manifestations that we as clinicians might use in our interpretation
of data, without going into possible specific mechanisms.
       In Figure 5.1 we see a number of possibilities for sur-
vival. Survival provides an explicit, well-defined end
point, and, of all living beings, man is the only one that
can see into the future, can plan and foresee his own demise.
Awareness and fear of death has been an overriding factor
in man's thoughts and anxieties and basis for much that is
apparent in social organizations, religion, philosophy, and
many areas of human activity. The biggest problem is survival. If we are to assume that all deaths are due to
environmental assault, and if we have a cohort which is born
in an environment that is totally benign, in which there is
no danger from the environment, then every individual that
is born should survive indefinitely (curve 1A). If we introduce risks into that environment, the risk would have a
certain, fairly constant ratio over a long period of historic
time. For instance, if there is a severe environment and
there is a 50% loss in the first unit of time, another 50%
in the second, another 50% in the third, etc., the survival

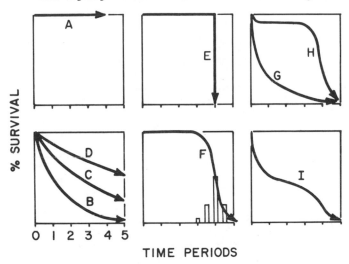

% SURVIVAL

0 1 2 3 4 5

TIME PERIODS

Figure 5.1

Theoretical patterns of survival. A: Infinite
survival in the absence of environmental hazards.
B: Death due to a constant rate of environmental
hazard. C, D: Decreased, but constant, levels of
environmental hazard. E: Survival, with death due
to precisely timed intrinsic mechanism. F: Intrinsically regulated survival with a distribution of
times of death. G: Survival related to external
hazards, with accelerated risk in infancy and childhood. H: Survival related to intrinsic factors, with
early losses due to inadequate development.
I: Survival related to all of the above factors.

curve would look something like Figure 1B if all deaths were
due to environmental hazards. On the other hand, as environment is improved, we would expect to see curves of the same
general convexity downward, but with more shallow slopes
so that survival of members of a cohort would be longer.
This is one possibility. This seems to be the one we
philosophically favor, because this implies that we can alter
the environment and, therefore, move this curve upward (1C
and 1D).

There are other possibilities. In mid-September few
leaves have turned color, but, in a few weeks more, leaves
will become red and then brown and finally drop off; eventually trees will be bare. There is a program for duration
of life for each leaf. The program may be very precise,
proceed so long, and then all individuals in the cohort will
suddenly cease to exist (1E). Or, there may be a distribution; some of the leaves have less vitality and are falling

off now, some will fall off in the next couple of weeks, most
will fall off in a month, and a few will straggle, and we'll
get a cohort survival curve that looks something like
Figure 1F.

   We have assumed that the newborn individual has the same
ability to cope with the environment as an older individual.
But if the newborn individual does not, then that newborn
individual may have an accelerated rate of loss until survivors adapt to a more mature curve after a period of time
(1G). On the other hand, there may be some individuals who
are not properly formed, who have birth defects and die
early, and then, at that point, we pick up curve 1H. Or we
may have a curve which incorporates all of these possibilities
(1I).

SURVIVORSHIP WHITE WOMEN

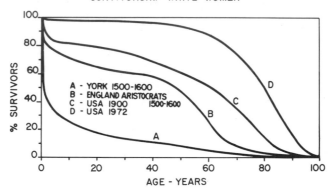

Figure 5.2

Actual patterns of survival. A: Women in the city
of York, England, sixteenth century (compare with
5.1G). B: English aristocrats, sixteenth century.
C: White women, USA, 1900 (compare B and C with
5.1I). D: White women, USA, 1972 (compare with
5.1H). Curves A and B adapted from Ursula Cowgill,
Sci. Amer. 222:104, 1970, and curves C and D from
Statistical Abstracts of the United States, 1975.
(Reprinted from Goldman, R. "Aging and Geriatric
Medicine," in Cecil Textbook of Medicine, 1979 ed.,
edited by P. B. Beeson, W. McDermott, and James B.
Wyngaarden, by permission of the publisher, W. B.
Saunders).

   Figure 5.2 shows what we actually see in human survival.
About five centuries ago in the city of York, England, survivorship for women looked something like the bottom curve.
The population of York during this century could not have
been maintained were it not for the people who moved in from

the countryside. In the first year, 55% of the girl babies
died. Only 18% lived to age 20, 11% to age 40, and 3 or 4%
to age 65. There was little need for geriatrics in this
population. The second curve represents aristocrats and,
probably, countryside in general. This curve resembles the
curve in Figure 1H which incorporates all of the elements.
It is the usual curve which is seen in nature. The next
curve is for white women in the United States in 1900. The
top curve represents the current situation in the United
States and it is almost identical for all developed countries.
This curve appears to represent an environment that has relatively little impact on survival, which seems to be controlled
primarily by intrinsic factors.

     If we wonder why we call ourselves civilized, this is
as good a reason as any. If we look at this curve, instead
of having only 11% of the white women survive to age 40, it
is now 95%; 82% will reach age 65; about two-thirds will
reach age 75, and one-third will reach age 85. The 85-year-
old group is our most rapidly increasing group today. We
don't have the wastage of life we had in the past. Survival
curves have shown continuous improvement up to the present.
If the environment is doing us in, there is no evidence of
it so far. This does not mean we don't have to be on guard,
but it does mean nothing has happened so far that has
reversed the trend. Again, this curve has the pattern in
which the environment has minimal influence and intrinsic
factors of survival have maximum influence. From theoretical
data we are not going to be able to improve the curve much
further unless we can slow the actual process of aging.

     Let us examine some of the theoretical considerations.
Figure 5.3A shows a curve which demonstrates the number of
deaths per thousand population at each age; age-specific
death rate. There is a fairly high infantile death rate
during the first year, but this drops rapidly to a low point
at about puberty, then the risk of dying goes up rather
steeply. In Figure 5.3B we see what happens if we plot age
on regular rectangular coordinates and death rate on log
coordinates. Notice that after a high infant mortality,
a low pubertal mortality, and some irregularity in early
adulthood, the risk increases as a straight line. Throughout the ages encompassed by the straight-line portion of the
curve, the risk of death at any given age is a function of
that age, not of any specific cause of death. Age is the
most important determinant of risk of dying in a given
environment. This is known as Gompertz Law, after an
English insurance actuary who first proposed it in 1825.
It has been keeping Lloyds of London in business for 150
years; biologists just found out about it. As we improve
the environment, we improve survival most in youth, but
we don't improve it so much in later life.

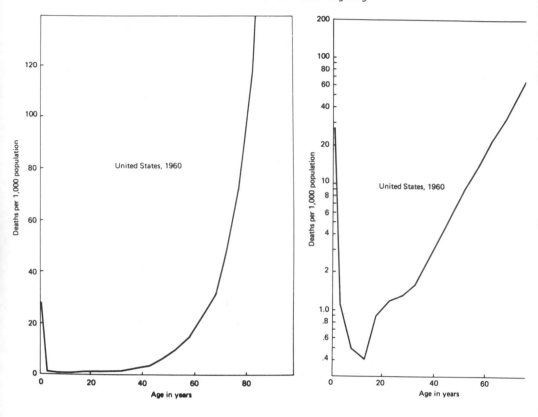

Figure 5.3A   Figure 5.3B

Risk of death at various ages in the United States, 1960. In 5.3A risk
is plotted on a rectangular scale, in 5.3B risk is plotted on a logarith-
mic scale.   (Reprinted from Fox, J. P., C. E. Hall, and L. R. Elveback,
Epidmiology, Man and Disease, © Copyright, The Macmillan Company,
1970, by permission of the publisher.)

     To show this in more specific terms, data for Swedish
women from 1750 to 1950 are presented in Figure 5.4. As the
environment has improved, the risk of a 13-year-old Swedish
girl not reaching age 14 decreased from seven in a thousand
(1750) to about six-tenth in a thousand (1950). In other
words, a little bit more than a tenfold improvement in two
centuries. But it has had very little effect in old age.
If they survive to age 85, the risk is essentially unchanged.

Figure 5.4

Death rates of
Swedish women from
1751 to 1950.
(Reprinted from
Jones H. B., in
Handbook of Aging
and the Individ-
ual: Psychological
and Biological
Aspects, edited by
James E. Birren,
© 1959 by The
University of
Chicago, by per-
mission of the
University of
Chicago Press.

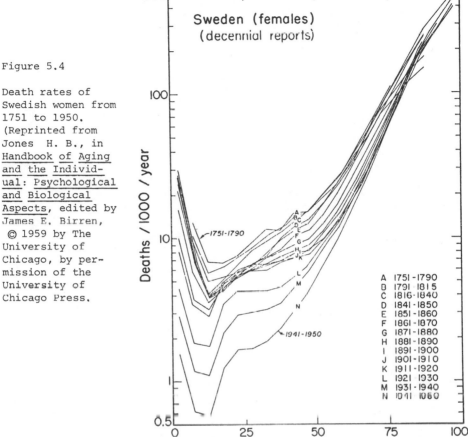

Sweden (females)
(decennial reports)

A	1751-1790
B	1791-1815
C	1816-1840
D	1841-1850
E	1851-1860
F	1861-1870
G	1871-1880
H	1881-1890
I	1891-1900
J	1901-1910
K	1911-1920
L	1921-1930
M	1931-1940
N	1941-1950

        So much for the Gompertz concept. Since there is a
geometric increase, what begins as a low risk of death in
early life continuously increases so that in very late life
it becomes extremely high. In 1867 Makeham, also a British
actuary, brought forth another concept, that if a constant
value is assigned to the risks of the environment and this
is added to the Gompertz formula, the resultant curves would
look like Figure 5.5. The more the environmental risk, the
higher the environmental component would be. If environmental
component is added to Gompertz component early in life, the
Gompertz component is so small that the sum of the two isn't
much more than the environmental factor alone. Only when the
individual becomes fairly advanced in age does the sum of the

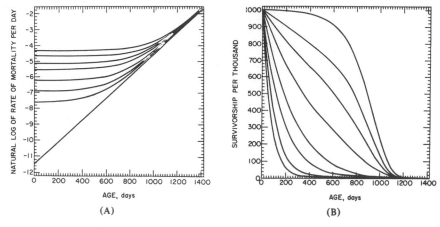

Figure 5.5

A: Age-specific death rates combining the intrinsic (age-independent) component with different levels of extrinsic (age-independent) risk. B: Survival curves derived from these rates: the upper curves of A (high environmental risk) are associated with the lower curves of B (low survival). (From HANDBOOK OF THE BIOLOGY OF AGING edited by C. E. Finch and L. Hayflick © 1977 by Litton Educational Publishing, Inc. Reprinted by permission of D. Van Nostrand Company.)

start drifting upward, and, of course, the larger the environmental factor, the later it is still evident. At advanced age the Gompertz component is so large that it obscures the environmental component, especially if the latter is relatively small. This resembles what we see. The top curve is the one in which the environmental factor is high; the bottom one is one in which the environmental factor is very small and the intrinsic component, as defined by the Gompertz formula, is dominant.

Although risks may be appearing at a constant rate, response to risks may be different. For instance, the first exposure to diptheria results in death or recovery; from then on the individual is immune. So, although exposure to diptheria may occur once every ten years, there is no risk at the second exposure. Trauma is another risk that is age related. Youths and young adults are notoriously reckless and unskilled, and accidental deaths tend to concentrate at this age. Risks of childbirth, both to the fetus and to the mother, have an interesting interaction. As infant mortality decreases, women need bear fewer children in order to maintain a zero population growth. Therefore, the risks of maternity are decreased not only because of improved general environment and technology, but also because of reduced frequency of childbirth risk. These environmental risks have all been reduced after early childhood. Additionally, one important cause of improved longevity is our increased knowledge of nutrition. The reduction of malnutrition and

of infection, our better ability to manage trauma and child-
birth--both for the child and for the mother--have greatly
reduced the risk of death in early life.

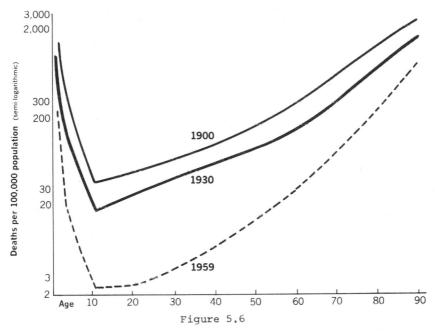

Figure 5.6

Age and mortality rates from pneumococcus pneumonia.
(From Reimann, H. A., Geriatrics 18:432-43, 1963.
Reprinted with permission of Geriatrics.)

Figure 5.6 shows the risk of dying of pneumococcus
pneumonia. Pneumococcus pneumonia is an acute illness, precisely diagnosed, and the patient recovers or dies. In 1900
there was a high juvenile and infantile mortality, a low
mortality in early adolescence, and then a rising mortality
in Gompertz fashion. Pneumonia is an acute episode, and yet
response to it is very age related. Between 1900 and 1930,
there was little improvement. Patients were moved to hospitals, got better nursing care, and might have received
oxygen. Then, between 1934 and 1943, pneumococcus antiserum,
sulfa drugs, and, finally, penicillin were introduced. By
1960 the risk had been almost entirely eliminated in adolescence, but there had been a smaller improvement at both age
extremes. Individuals respond to an acute stress in an age-
related manner that resembles the Gompertz curve for all
causes of deaths.

Figure 5.7 shows age-specific mortal risk for four most
common causes of death. Risk of dying of heart disease and

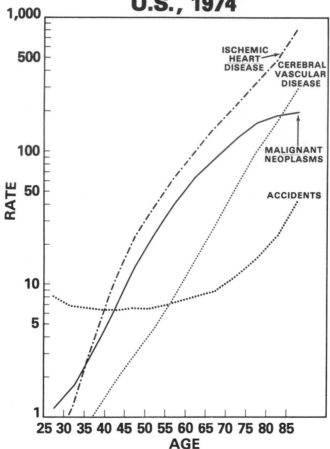

Figure 5.7

Age-specific mortality rates for the four commonest causes
of death. Plotted from Vital Statistics of the U.S., 1975.

of stroke each increase linearly on a semi-log plot. Risk
of dying of cancer also increases with age, but not quite
linearly. The risk in any one year of dying of any one
of these three diseases continues to increase, so that if
the individual escapes from one cause, there is a rapidly
increasing risk from one of the others. Accidents are
environmental, and it is interesting that between the age
25 and age 55 there is very little change in accident mortality, only the difference between six and eight for ten
thousand male population per year for the 30 year span.
After age 55 mortality rate increases and approaches linear-
ity. The reason is not that older people have more accidents,
but when they have an accident they have a declining ability
to recover. This is the classic combination of environmental
risk combined with intrinsic debility.
     We have seen that there are environmental factors and
there are intrinsic factors. These interact in varying
proportions to affect survival. Now, intrinsic factors
appear to be overwhelmingly most important. The major
problem of gerontology and aging has been differentiation
of normal from disease phenomena. If the patient has pneumonia, he has an infiltrate in the lung, there are organisms
in the sputum, there is fever, and leukocytosis, and other
manifestations of the disease. Pneumonia is a specific
entity that is either present or absent. But we see a
progression in the frequency of certain chronic disorders
with age. Is this a manifestation of age itself, or is it
a disease? Does one person have a weakness in one organ
system and another have a weakness in another organ system,
and therefore do these manifest differently with age?

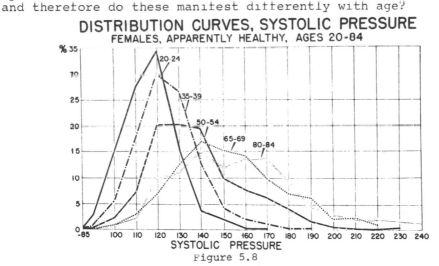

DISTRIBUTION CURVES, SYSTOLIC PRESSURE
FEMALES, APPARENTLY HEALTHY, AGES 20-84

Figure 5.8

Distribution of systolic blood pressures, by age, in
U.S. women. (Note that there is no abrupt separation of
hypertensive from non-hypertensive individuals.)

Is that why we age differently? Figure 5.8 shows range
of systolic blood pressures for women by age, but men are
similar. There is a normal distribution. Blood pressure
goes up with age, so that by age 65, 50% have a blood pressure above 150 systolic which is arbitrarily well into the
hypertensive range. We do not have a group that are normal
and a group that are abnormal, we have a continuity. There
are some people in whom the hypertension is due to a specific cause, such as kidney disease and certain endocrine
diseases. But most individuals have a distribution of
height and weight. They don't all have the same blood
pressure. We speak of normal and abnormal blood pressure.
But what does that mean?

Table 5.1.   Relative risk of death related to blood pressure

Systolic B.P.	Mortality ratio %	Diastolic B.P.	Mortality ratio%
88 - 97	78	48 - 67	83
98 - 127	88	68 - 82	97
128 - 137	118	83 - 87	129
138 - 147	155	88 - 92	150
148 - 157	194	93 - 97	188
158 - 167	244	98 - 102	234
168 - 177	242	103 - 112	262

Source: From 1959 build and blood pressure study, Society of Actuaries.
Note: Mortality ratio (percent) of actual to expected mortality
   according to systolic and diastolic levels (males, policy issue ages
   15 to 69).

Let us relate blood pressure to risk of dying. Table
5.1 shows the relative risk of death related to blood pressure. Notice that there is no point where there is a plateau
in the risk. The lower the blood pressure, the longer the
survival, and the higher it is, the greater the risk. In
other words. we cannot pick any point and say arbitrarily
that above is disease, below is not. All we can say is
that relatively one is better off if blood pressure is low,
and worse off if blood pressure is high.
     Figure 5.9 demonstrates risk factors. They are distri-
butional, with frequencies represented on the lower curve.
They may be blood cholesterol levels, blood sugar levels,
blood pressures, uric acid levels, or any others, identified
or unidentified. We could probably find more if we started
looking at them. The upper curve is the average risk of
death correlated with risk factor. The left side is the

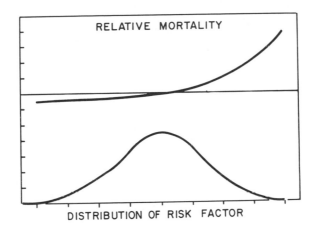

Figure 5.9

The relationship of individual risk factor status
to mortal risk.

favorable side of the risk factor and risk of death decreases.
On the right side, it increases. But where is normal and
Where is abnormal? Is somebody with a blood pressure of 139
normal, but with 141 abnormal? In other words, we are talking
about what might be called quantitative disease. There are
many situations in which this concept is applicable.

A heart beats 70 times a minute, 1440 minutes a day,
365 days a year, 70 years on the average. With each beat,
blood vessels expand and contract. Walls of blood vessels
contain collagen and elastin. Once collagen is deposited,
it stays in place for a lifetime. Collagen has only limited
capability of restoration. Elastin also changes with age.
Let us imagine that the blood vessels expand and contract
with each heartbeat and they have a level of damage, which
is repaired to a certain extent after each beat. If the
individual has hypertension and the heart pounds away at the
blood vessels, the response will be more abrupt, more dam-
aging. It is possible that the cumulative damage with age
may be accelerated as a result. What we see is the acute
stroke, the acute heart attack. We don't see the progressive change in blood vessels that leads to that acute attack.
We see only acute manifestations of chronic, long-term
change. It is possible many things that we call diseases
are merely manifestations of aging at different rates in
different organ systems. It remains to be seen, but evidence is increasing that can be interpreted in this way.

Most of us would like to believe we reach maturity and
nothing happens to us from then on. That if it weren't for
the slings and arrows of fate, we would go on with our youth
pattern forever, and if we could only hold back the forces
of environment, we could hold back old age. Biologically,
this is probably not the case. We must take an entirely
different look at the problem.

Let us turn to Figure 5.2. All the data seem to imply
that whatever is the matter with the environment now, it has
less effect on us than it has ever had before. More importantly, if 96% of white women live to age 40, what changes
to the system will improve it to that point? We have only
a narrow 4% gap for improvement, at least in terms of survivorship, but the potential for worsening the system is
infinitely greater. In other words, it behooves us to be
certain that we know what we are doing before changes are
made. The 4% may be due to a number of causes. Some may
be the result of rapid traumatic incidents, such as explo-
sions or crashes, which preclude rescue or treatment. Some
might be due to diseases or conditions for which we don't
yet have treatment. Some might be due to an error on the part
of the health facility professional once we got there. Some
may be due to inaccessibility of care. At least four causes
for 4%. This doesn't allow much room for change. It seems
to me that we cannot reduce the gap by using less well
trained professionals. The present level of performance
has been the result of increasing knowledge, skill and,
technology. If there is an argument for improved access,
logic should dictate that it continue in this direction.

This presentation is a basis for thinking about dynamics
of the aging process. It is a process; it is within all of
us; it is interacted upon by the environment. This shouldn't
create any sense of hopelessness. As physicians, we try to
identify the abnormal and make it normal. We have gone almost
as far as we can with that approach. If we are to prolong
life further, we must find the normal and modify it, to
make it abnormal in a favorable direction. It is a different approach, but it is the one to which we must be dedicated if we are to make significant progress in the future.

CHAPTER 6

OUR FUTURE SELVES

George L. Maddox

In 1976 the United States proudly celebrated the 200th anniversary of a successful revolution. Less obvious and less
noted were three other revolutions:
   1. A demographic revolution characterized by a dramatic change in the age structure of our population;
   2. A related confrontation challenging existing social
arrangements for meeting personal and social needs; and
   3. An emerging revolution in individual and public
imagery of what late life is and can be.

A Demographic Revolution

The demographic facts about the changing age composition in
our population are clear. The proportion of older people,
those age 65 and over, has doubled in this century and will
increase from 10% to perhaps 17% early in the next century.
One-third of the 23 million older persons are "very old"
(over age 75) and one in ten are age 85 or older.
   At mid-decade average life expectancy at birth in the
United States was about 72 years, 69 for males and 76 for
females. This gender difference produces a skewed male/
female distribution in later years. For example, at age 85
females outnumber males more than two to one.
   While average life expectancy is increasing, the length
of the life span has increased little. Actuaries continue
to consider life beyond age 94 as a statistically rare
event.
   The increasing number of older persons in our population
reflects not extensions of the life span but the increased
probability of living into the later years. At mid decade,
74% of persons born can expect to survive to age 65, and
then to live 16 years longer; 52% can expect to achieve 75
years, then live 10 years longer; 23% will achieve 85 years,
and then live six years longer.
   If we add to the conventionally old and very old populations the "young old" (age 55 to 60), the older population
of the nation essentially doubles--46 million persons and
20% of the total.

A Revolutionary Challenge to Social Institutions

The consequences of growing old are not altogether benign.
An aging population is at increased risk for illness, impairment, poverty, and social isolation. About 80% of older
persons have at least one chronic condition and about 20%
have a chronic condition which impairs their ability to

carry out usual social roles without help. Five percent are
in long-term care institutions and a majority of these are
severely impaired and dependent; at least another 5%-8%
who live in the community are also severely impaired and
dependent. While most older persons are not accurately
characterized in such negative terms, the demand for health
and social services increases with age. The average health
cost per capita of persons age 65 and over at mid-decade was
$1,360, about three times higher than the cost for adults
generally. Various health and social support programs for
older persons currently cost $112 billion--or 5% of the Gross
National Product and a significant increase in cost is forecast for the decades ahead. Two-thirds of the health costs
in later life are purchased with public dollars, although
older persons contribute to the public funds utilized.
The important points to keep in mind are that the requirements for health and social services change with age; the
age composition of our population is shifting dramatically
toward the upper range of age; therefore, a challenge to
existing social arrangements for meeting our national wants and
needs follows. For instance, the news media also understand
the following challenges that are as current as the morning
newspaper.

Income Maintenance

The architects of Social Security built a politically and
economically viable system in 1935 that has served us well.
Social Security was never intended to provide for all the
economic needs of the retired, widowed, and disabled. Nor
could they have anticipated the high rate of survival of the
"very old," an economy characterized by inflation and unemployment, and the popularity of early retirement. The
evidence is now clear. Today 25% of older persons live in
or near poverty. Adequately secured income in late life
is going to cost us as much as 250%-300% more in the next
several decades.

Health Care

Modern high-technology medicine concentrated in medical center hospitals has performed miracles. As one might expect,
miracles have a high price tag. At the same time, preventive
care, primary care, and community-based care have languished.
Less than 1% of Medicare funds, e.g., are used to purchase
community-based services. Long-term institutional care has
earned a reputation for high cost and variable quality.
There are over 22,000 nursing homes with over a million beds
occupied mostly by older persons at a cost of over $10
billion annually. Professional schools, particularly medical schools, have done little to teach students about, much
less to motivate them toward, geriatric care. The continuing

neglect of gerontological and geriatric training in professional education generally is remarkable in light of the
demand for health care.

Transportation

The love affair between Americans and their private automobiles continues despite escalating cost and decreasing resources for energy. This love affair has permitted and
encouraged suburbanization, an intended separation of
individuals from their places of work and an unintended
separation from sources of services. We centralize services
for reasons of economy and professional convenience and
assume that persons, however remote geographically, will get
to them. Public transportation is not a high priority. And
never mind that some individuals do not have or cannot use
private transportation--the poor, the impaired, the elderly.
When older people are asked to specify their special areas
of want or need, they place transportation high on the list.
We are aware that getting people in rural areas and services
together is a difficult and unsolved problem. We are only a
few years away from the realization that "the suburban
problem" will be added to "the rural problem." There are a
growing number of impaired older persons without private
transportation in our suburbs, where health and social services are not located. The U.S. General Accounting Office
in Cleveland, Ohio, has recently documented that impaired
older persons in the central city are more likely to receive
needed services than are equally impaired older persons in
the suburbs.

Education

For years we have proudly given "terminal degrees" to adolescents and young adults. Institutions of higher education
have looked with suspicion, occasionally with contempt, at
adult and continuing education. Learning is a lifetime
affair! How convenient it has been to assume that older
people neither want nor are capable of continued learning.
How convenient it has been to assume that a professional
diploma frees one from the need of continuing education. We
are beginning to have second thoughts about the wisdom of
giving anyone, especially a professional person, a terminal
degree. That appears to be dangerous as well as unwise.

An Emerging Revolution of Imagery and Expectations

The less obvious but important revolution to be considered
is a revolution in our thinking about late life, what is it
and what it might be. Science has contributed in important
ways. Research at the Duke University Center for the Study
of Aging and Human Development provides an illustration.

Almost a quarter century ago, biomedical, behavioral, and
social scientists like Philip Handler, E. W. Busse, William
Anlyan, Juanita Kreps, and Joseph Spengler anticipated many
of the important personal and societal issues that an aging
population would produce and mobilized the resources of a
great university to address them systematically. Duke's
longitudinal studies have documented, for example, about
30,000 years in the lives of middle aged and older individuals who experience relatively normal, satisfying, and satisfactory lives in one or another community. This research
has pioneered a new realistic image of what it means to grow
older. This image stresses:

Variety

People do not become more alike as they age. Older people
have different styles, different values, different needs, and
different wants.

Continuity

Late life presents challenges but not many surprises. Middle
aged individuals who do not cope with challenges well, do not
like their work, are threatened by illness or death, and do
not like their children, tend to become older people who do
not cope well, do not like retirement, are threatened by
illness or death, and have unsatisfying relationships with
their children. Most older people manage the crisis of life
transitions very well. And that includes retirement, death
of spouse, illness, and the departure of children from home.

Unused Potential

Most individuals do not live up to their physical, intellectual, or moral potential on a day-to-day basis. In heroic
moments most of us manage to demonstrate reserves of energy
and resourcefulness we hoped and perhaps suspected we had.
Research at Duke has demonstrated the importance of distin-
guishing aging and illness. Illness and excessive dependency
are correlates of age. But at least 6 out of 10 older persons
are free of impairments which require special help from
others. Significant loss of reality orientation, or dementia,
from whatever cause, is the probable experience of only 5 in
100 persons over age 65 and the probability increases only
to 20 in 100 for persons over age 80. In the absence of
serious debilitating illness, intellectual capacity measured
in adulthood is maintained well into the 70's. Any physical
capacity can be significantly improved by appropriate
training at any age   Dr. Richard Rahe, a medical research
scientist in the U.S. Navy, argues that for a wide range of
older persons physiological capacity can be significantly
increased. The average person's measured physiological performance tends to decrease by about 1% per year in later life.

Later life is a time characterized by unused but mobilizable
reserves of intellectual and physical energy.

Environmental Opportunity

Everyone knows that children and young people have to have
opportunities to grow and to develop their potential. Does
everyone know that this is also true of older people? What
we see in the behavior of older people is probably as much or
more a commentary on those of us who are responsible for
environmental opportunities than a commentary on older people. Disengaged, uninvolved older people tend to be found
in communities providing limited opportunities for older
people to be involved in community life. Is anyone surprised by that?
    The revolution in consciousness of older people about
themselves parallels the revolution in scientific thought
about late life. More and more individuals are arriving at
old age with a reasonably secure income, adequate health, a
record of political participation, and the expectation of
remaining socially active and of having their wants and needs
taken seriously. Older people are more politically active
than individuals in their twenties, a fact suggesting that
the wants and perceived needs of older people will get the
attention of the legislators. Active older people have
learned an important lesson about political effectiveness
in a society that operates on the principle of "interest
group liberalism." Organize! While we have not developed
a "politics of age," the potential for political confrontation over age-related issues is considerable if communities
ignore the rising self-consciousness of older Americans.
Fortunately, older voters in the United States now provide
a relatively rare illustration of political altruism; that
is, their self-interest tends to be tempered with an awareness of the needs of future generations.
    Older people are not problems, they have problems.
Some of those problems are created by us through the attitudes we have as professionals and as citizens who make
political decisions about how the goods, services, and opportunities of communities will be distributed. Moreover, their
problems of income, health care, transportation, and learning
will be our problems soon unless institutional change is
achieved.
    This is why, in the lives of those who are currently
old, we see our future selves. When the National Institute
on Aging (N.I.A.) was created as the newest program in the
National Institutes of Health in 1975, the Congress required
a five-year plan that would specify the work to be done. As
a member of the National Advisory Council of N.I.A., I recall vividly outlining the challenges of later life and the
biomedical, behavioral, and social scientific research, the
basic research and clinical training, and the demonstrations

in new and effective ways to deliver services needed to
respond to these challenges. We were not addressing the
problems of some faceless, nameless older people. We were
planning for our world, our fate, our future selves.

Realistic Optimism about the Future of Aging

The genius of this nation lies in a fundamental sense of
fairness, a commitment to pragmatic solutions, and a deep
faith that we can make rather than simply endure history.
There are many signs for optimism about the future of aging
in this country.

Government is responding at many levels and in some useful ways. There have been three White House Conferences on
Aging. There is a National Institute on Aging; a Center for
the Study of the Mental Health of the Elderly in the National
Institute of Mental Health; an Older Americans Act; an
Administration on Aging; Medicare and Medicaid; special committees on aging in both houses of Congress; and a network
of services for older persons in every state and in most
communities. These developments are not the solution to
problems related to aging. They are positive signs of sub-
stantial and relevant public response.

Professional organizations are beginning to respond in
relevant ways. The Institute of Medicine, National Academy
of Sciences, has issued an excellent report on the steps
necessary to reduce unnecessary dependence in later life and
also a report recommending guidelines for developing medical
education in geriatric care. Professional societies are
regularly including gerontological and geriatric topics in
their programs and offering continuing education opportunities
The Geronotological Society has an active membership of 5,000
and is growing. Regional and state gerontological societies
are proliferating. A professional is less likely, when faced
with an older client with a problem, to say, "What do you
expect at your age?" If the uninformed professional asks
such a question, the probability of a challenge is increasingly likely from the lay as well as the professional community. Therapeutic optimism is increasingly the rule and
such optimism underlies a new and realistic basis for intervention in the interest of maintaining appropriate independence in late life. Optimism on the part of those who work
with older persons in the hope of preventing and minimizing
impairments and unnecessary dependency is not based on the
denial of the real losses that are inevitably associated
sooner or later in life. After all, life has a common
outcome. But the pathways to that outcome are demonstrably
varied and modifiable until the evidence is otherwise.
Therapeutic optimism is based on the experience of an
increasing number of clinicians who have demonstrated their
ability to increase the capacity of impaired older people
for appropriate independent living. A good rule for any

clinician working with older people is to demonstrate rather
than assume that an impairment is unmodifiable. More and
more medical schools, as well as professional schools, are
providing new opportunities for discovering the satisfaction
of experiencing the difference the application of that rule
can make in the life of an older person. Some medical faculty
members say that medical students are not interested in geriatrics. There is evidence that this is an uninformed opinion. At Duke we know there is student interest.

Our options for securing adequate income in the increasing number of years in retirement are not attractive but they
are clear. Social Security does not provide the sole source
of income in retirement and will not do so in the years ahead,
even with the increases in taxes already forecast. Private
pensions and personal financial assets will continue to be
important unless and until a decision is made to redistri-
bute income over the life-cycle through taxation on income
in the adult years many times higher than the social security
taxes currently paid or contemplated for the future. We must
rethink our retirement policy which currently encourages
early departure from work. The minimum retirement age at
which full social security benefits would be paid could be
raised from 65 to 68. However, despite the fact that recent
legislation has raised the age of mandatory retirement from
65 to 70, a legal victory for older persons, the continued
preference of most older persons in the United States is for
earlier retirement.

Learning as a lifetime activity is being rediscovered.
A year ago the Institute for Learning in Retirement was
created at Duke University. Similar developments are evident in many institutions of higher education and in many
communities as the interests in and capacity for lifetime
learning among older persons have become more apparent. Lifetime learning means many things to older people. For some,
continued learning is an end in itself. For others, it is an
avenue to a new career as a paid worker or as a volunteer in
the community. There is one potential benefit of learning
as a lifetime affair that tends to be overlooked. Adults
have found it easy to disidentify with schools and the support
of public education when the education of their own children
is completed. This would be a less likely outcome if schools
were for everyone in the community and not just for children.
A community school can claim and expect community support.

A Question of Values

What is the national intent and will regarding late life?
What is our future? During the national celebration of our
aging nation in 1976 I imagined some future archaeologist
rummaging in our junk heaps the way current archaeologists
rummage in the junk heaps of Greece, Rome, and Jerusalem
for clues about the life-styles of peoples and nations.

Future archaeologists trying to understand us might be intrigued by the labels on the bottles we are leaving behind as possible clues about our values. What would be made of phrases like "No Deposit--No Return," "Dispose of Properly," and "Return for Refill"?

These labels reflect real differences in attitudes and options involving people as well as things. Do we really intend that people in our affluent society have the juice sucked out and be thrown away? Do we intend simply to dispose of them properly? Or do we intend to make it possible to return and return and return for refill?

I know what I want for my future self. What about you?

CHAPTER 7

EVALUATION AND PLACEMENT

R. Knight Steel

Placement is the process of choosing a living situation most suitable to the individual. The term implies that there are multiple alternatives, for without such options the index person would just have to make do. Historically, placement became a concern only when facilities other than the home came into existence and when society decided against the extended family and sanctioned the very process of placement.

The physician is the gatekeeper in our health system. This professional prescribes not only drugs and procedures but often the living situation for many of us as we get older and as we become more dependent for support in our daily existences on both other persons and the system. In discussing placement, this model of the physician as gatekeeper will be used permitting us to look at: (1) the placee, or patient; (2) the gatekeeper, or the physician; (3) the gate and its lock; and (4) the building inside the gate.

Three observations will serve as background. First, it is important to get a sense of the magnitude of institutional care (1). Now, there are in excess of a million long-term-care beds in the United States, a number that equals or exceeds the number of acute care beds. At least 90% of these beds are occupied by the elderly. This represents 5% of the 22 million elderly. However, as persons are discharged or die, these beds are filled by others. This means that about 20% of all of us at all ages will at one time or another pass through such institutions by whatever name they are called. Over the past 10 to 15 years there has been a decrease in the number of mental hospital beds in this country and an even greater rise in the number of nursing home beds. Many of the elderly have been moved from one to the other, with the result that this process of placement has become more complicated.

Also, we will present a few thoughts on aging and disease and what this means to the aging population. The geriatrician states emphatically that the process of aging is different from the sheer accumulation of disease. Over time we all age, and the longer we survive, the greater the likelihood we have of accumulating chronic illnesses. Thus, the majority of those over 65 years of age carry with them one or more chronic conditions. Many have some limitation of activities due to the superimposition of these diseases on the process of aging, a physiologic phenomenon not in itself limiting to the performance of our usual activities, but one that limits our reserve and our endurance. Eighty-five

percent of the elderly manage quite well with few, if any,
support services other than routine care and occasional
medical intervention. These figures are misleading as they
reflect only one moment in time, and as was seen to be true
with nursing home utilization, the process is dynamic.
Thus, more than 15% of the elderly will require services at
one time or another so as to remain at home or at the lowest
possible level of care. Often this need is temporary as
the person either recovers over a period of time or dies.
     These figures about the well elderly are also misleading.
The elderly account for only 10.9% of our population now (2)
and will account for about 12% of our population by the turn
of the century. Within this segment of America, there are
the "young old," those ages 65 to 75, and the "old old,"
those 75 years of age and older. Since the definition of
the "old old" vs. those whose life has spanned at least 65
years dates from Baron Von Bismark and is an arbitrary, non-
physiologic breakpoint in the life span, it is not surprising
that those ages 65 to 75 differ remarkably little from those
ages 45 to 65. At about age 75 the accumulation of disease,
in addition to limitations associated with the process of
aging, produces functional disabilities of major proportions
in a sizable percent of this group of the "old old." It is
this very old and relatively very infirm population who
suffer disproportionately from pathological conditions and
who utilize our health care resources to the greatest extent
on a per capita basis. It is this "old old" group of persons that is the fastest growing segment of our population.
     Thirdly, it must be emphasized that the elderly arrive
at the "gate" and seek the help of a "gatekeeper" as a rule
only at times of desperation. Elaine Brody at the Philadelphia Geriatric Center has gathered data which clearly demonstrate that, under most circumstances, families make every
effort to care for their older members (3). They seek alternate placement for them only when they reach the breaking
point, financially, emotionally, and physically. The myth
that families dump their elder members is exactly that, a
myth!
     A moment's reflection about persons residing in insti-
tutions will support this contention. The mean age of persons in nursing homes is in excess of 80 years in many
settings. The elderly population is lopsided with respect
to the sexes. For all those age 65 and older, there are
only 69 males for every 100 females and this ratio of males
to females decreases to 58 per 100 by age 75 and still further to 50 per 100 by age 85. Furthermore, only 39% of
all older women are married in contrast to 79% of all older
men: by age 75 only 1 in 4 women is married (4). Because
of the striking difference in life expectancy between the
sexes many of these elderly women, if they had male chil-
drer, have seen their children die. For white females the

death rate between 65 and 74 is only half of that for white
males. Thus, the residents of long-term care institutions
are predominantly women without spouses and often without
close relatives. These, then, are some of the demographic
and physiologic characteristics of the population who will
require placement.

Attention should be drawn to the serious problems facing
our middle-aged population in the 1980s. They
must now try to care for their elderly parents at the same
time that they struggle to understand their adolescent children while they proceed on through college; all occurring
during a time of inflation and a period of widening opportunities with concommitant demands especially on the middle-
aged women. This set of circumstances will increasingly
affect the need for placement.

There is nothing more important than a complete medical
evaluation of "the placee," or the patient prior to placement. This alone would facilitate the proper placement of
the majority of our elderly, not to mention the prevention
and treatment of considerable disease. After all, placement
is merely the determination of the needs of the elderly and
how and where those needs might be met most effectively and
efficiently.

There is described, in the Journal of the American
Medical Association, an evaluation and placement service in
Rochester, New York (5). Patients seeking placement in long-
term care facilities in Monroe County were seen by a physician for a complete history and physical examination and,
in addition, by a nurse with special competence in geriatrics
and knowledge about community services. After the patient
was seen and a routine set of laboratory data obtained, this
patient was "conferenced" by a doctor, a nurse, and a social
worker, who was invaluable in aiding in financial matters.
Sometimes, other nurses and professionals who had an interest
in this patient attended the meeting. A decision as to the
appropriate level of placement was made and then this decision was passed on to the family, the patient, and the
referring physician. Potential locations included (1) the
patient's home, perhaps with ancillary services, (2) a pro-
prietary home, (3) a health-related facility, (4) a nursing
home, (5) an acute hospital, (6) a rehabilitation service,
or, under rare circumstances, (7) a psychiatric unit. The
patient was seen after an interval of three months or so to
reevaluate the circumstances of placement even though the
patient has agreed to the level of care proposed. This permitted an opportunity to discuss once again any placement
concerns the patient or family related.

These authors discovered that less than one half of the
332 persons seen in the Evaluation and Placement Unit had a
personal physician whom they saw on a regular basis. Fifty-
five percent of cases seen and evaluated resulted in

recommendations for further diagnostic procedures, medical treatment, or rehabilitative efforts even before a final decision about placement could be made. "More specifically for 34% of all patients seen, a program of active medical treatment or a trial of intensive rehabilitation treatment was recommended and arranged for and for another 23%, more diagnostic medical studies were sought before a decision was made" (6).

In 1974 Steel, Williams, Fairbanks, and Knox reported on the review of only the laboratory data from 200 consecutive geriatric patients seen in an Evaluation and Placement Unit (7). Laboratory screening procedures consisted of a hemogram, urinanalysis, SMA 12, electrocardiogram (EKG), and chest roetgenogram. These findings are summarized in Table 7.1. Note the high percentage of abnormalities. By examining the charts and not including any information obtained from the history or the physical examination of the patient, a table (Table 7.2) of the most significant "Possible Diagnoses" was constructed. It is unlikely that any of the conditions were known to the patient, the patient's family, or the patient's physician, if one existed! This list of treatable conditions does not include large numbers of persons with some measure of renal insufficiency, an abnormal chest film or EKG if such variations from normal were judged most likely to be stable abnormalities. Such information would be important to any plan of management of these persons. Nor does this table include many findings such as hematuria, which would obviously require further study. It is important to remember that this patient sample was not drawn from Appalachia, but from those living in one of the richest counties in the United States, both in dollars and in the number of physicians in practice.

Let us assume that a complete medical evaluation has been undertaken, all treatable illnesses treated, and the patient's condition stabilized. In other words, total medical needs have been detailed and those readily treatable, treated. Those needs remaining so define the patient's medical condition that some sort of placement other than the usual setting is considered.

Regrettably, this methodical process all too often is not followed as the patient, in most occasions, is seen only when an acute illness intervenes or when the last straw is piled on an already overburdened camel. This may take the form of a close friend, who has always helped the patient, deciding to leave town, a precipitous increase in rent, or just plain exasperation on the part of the next of kin or the doctor, who almost invariably points the patient in the direction of some nursing home with the idea that this will solve the problem of the patient as well as that of the one doing the pointing.

The highest level of care is not necessarily the best.

Table 7.1 Laboratory Abnormalities Found in 200 Consecutive EPU Geriatric Patients

Item	Normal Range	Number of Abnormalities			
		High	Low	Total	Abnormal
SMA-12 Blood Chemical Tests (200 patients)					
Calcium	(9.0-10.5 mg/100 ml.)	2	12	14	7
Phosphorus	(2.5-4.5 mg/100 ml)	3	8	11	6
Alk. phosphatase	(30-85 IU)	89	–	89	45
Total protein	(6.0-8.0 gms)	4	4	8	4
Albumin	(3.5-5.0 gms)	–	12	12	6
Bilirubin	(0.2-1.0 mg/100 ml)	2	2	4	2
LDH	(100-225 IU)	13	–	13	7
SGOT	(<40IU)	13	–	13	7
Cholesterol	(150-300 mg/100 ml)	18	5	23	12
BUN	(<20 mg/100 ml)	78	–	78	39
Glucose	(see text)	46	2	48	24
Uric acid	(2.5-8.0 mg/100 ml)	15	2	17	9
Hematologic Tests (200 patients)					
Erythrocyte sed. rate	(>40 mm/hr)			44	22
Hematocrit	(<38%)			43	22
Leukocyte count	(<3000 or >12000/cu mm)	3	1	4	2
Urinalysis (160 patients)					
Albuminuria				21	13
Ketonuria				1	1
Hemoglobinuria				7	4
Other					
Electrocardiogram (198 patients)				158	79
Chest roetgenogram (195 patients)				141	72

Source: From Steel, K., Williams, T. F., Fairbank, M., and Knox, K. "Laboratory Screening in the Evaluation and Placement of Geriatric Patients." J. Am. Geriatr. Soc. 22:(12)539, 1974.

Table 7.2   The Most Significant "Possible Diagnoses" Indicated by Abnormalities Detected during Laboratory Screening

	Patients	Possible Diagnoses
1.	Female aged 81; Ca 5.2, P 5.2, BUN 23 (Mg/100 ml)	Secondary hypoparathyroidism
2.	Female aged 72; Ca 8.4, p 1.2 (mg/100 ml); Alk ptase >350 IU	Malabsorption
3.	Female aged 74; BUN 100, P 7.0 (mg/100 ml); Alk ptase >200 IU	Renal osteodystrophy
4.	Female aged 73; BUN 75 mg, Alb 3.4 gm (/100 ml); 3+ proteinuria	Glomerulitis
5.	Female aged 85; LDH 253 IV, MCV 127 cu ᵤ, Hcrit 34%	Pernicious anemia
6.	Female aged 97; Chol 148 mg/100 ml. Hcrit 31%, MCV 116 cu ᵤ, WBC 2800/cu mm	Malabsorption; folate or B-12 deficiency
7.	Male aged 80, Hcrit 20%	Found to have carcinoma of bowel
8.	Female aged 79; Hcrit 36%, MCV 71 cu ᵤ Alk ptase 143 IU	Gastointest. disease; possible neoplasia
9.	Female aged 68, blood glucose 57 mg/100 ml	Dumping syndrome due to subtotal gastrectomy
10-18.	Nine patients; blood glucose 207-500 mg/100 ml	Diabetes mellitus

Source: From Steel, K., Williams, T. F., Fairbank, M., and K. Knox. "Laboratory Screening in the Evaluation and Placement of Geriatric Patients." J. Am. Geriatr. Soc., 22:(12)542, 1974.

It may make the patient too dependent and too inactive and, of course, it is unduly expensive for the patient, the family, and society. The proper level of care is indeed the one that satisfies all of the major needs of the patient, no more and no less. In a study unique in its size and its thoroughness conducted in Monroe County, 25% of all nursing home patients were screened (8). Only 46.2% of such patients were found to be properly placed. 30.2% should have been at a lower level of care. This was the stimulus for the intro- duction of the Evaluation Placement Unit described previously.

Those patient needs that determine placement require emphasis. As stated by E. V. Morton and R. M. Tyndall: "Illness in the elderly has many unusual features. In no other group of patients does sickness so often occur as a result of a combination of physical, mental, and social fac- tors. It is a characteristic of geriatric medicine that the patient is at the same time often in need of medical, psychiatric, and social aid. The patient is confused because he is sick; and he is sick, in part at least, because he is neglected, lonely and often poor. All of these features of his illness require assessment, diagnosis, and treatment if he is to be made well and return to health and indepen- dence rather than left to degenerate into a state of chronic invalidism and often to remain unnecessarily occupying a hospital bed for many years, variously described as 'typical geriatric' or 'chronic sick'" (9). Those physicians who set up a Joint Assessment and Early Treatment Unit in institu- tions cannot help but influence practicing physicians about the processes of placement and the care of those so placed.

If we consider now the "gate and its lock," we must change directions slightly and get some additional background information. With the costs of health care rising at an annual rate between 12% and 14%, all third-party payers, including you and me, but most especially Washington, are considering how to control them. Therefore, the costs for our present and future health care system will double in five or six years and double again each five to six year period thereafter. In 1975, the total expenditure in the United States for health care was 118.5 billion dollars. Since then, it has risen by many tens of billions of dollars.

Those over age 65 make up only 10.9% of the population but account for 30% of these costs; and about 70% of this 30%, or more than a fifth, of all health care expenditures is expended on hospital and nursing home care for the elderly (10). This is all the more striking when one real- izes that long-term care, or other than acute hospital care, is not well covered by third-party payers. It is no wonder that planners are concerned about including long-term care costs in a national health program.

This statistical and fiscal information is essential to our understanding of the process of placement. It would be

naive to think that simply by determining the needs required
and what should be available with our present knowledge and
technology we can properly place a person. The key we pos-
sess may not enable us to enter the place we desire, as the
third-party payers simply change "locks" by adding restrictive guidelines for admission. Some are so limiting that
the requirements are essentially dictated by the "lockmaker"
and not the physician. This might be construed by some as
a way of practicing medicine without a license! In addition,
many a physician has been worn down by the inordinate amounts
of paper work and numbers of administrative contacts needed
to complete a placement process. Since most physicians in
practice do not employ a social worker, it is often impossible to find the proper placement for a patient because of
the time-consuming cost to complete such a processing.

Because of restrictive reimbursement policies by government agencies, the need for fiscal soundness and profit by
nursing homes, and for other reasons as well, most long-
term care institutions are loathe to take on the management
of more than a few patients who might require undue quantities of time and effort on the part of the nursing staff.
Thus, there is a tendency for the placer, or his or her
appointee, to scatter among different homes a number of
seriously ill patients who require considerable care.

Lastly, we come to the "building inside the gate."
First, the setting chosen should offer neither too few nor
too many services, both extremes being detrimental to
patient care and personal well-being. Although, in reality,
limited choices are available and compromise may be necessary, all of us should be encouraged to participate in our
own care and be master of our own souls as much as possible.
Also, although strictly medical needs may of necessity dictate placement, it must never be forgotten that the location
chosen is more than a "bed." It is a residence. The facility should be evaluated in terms of human services as well
as medical ones. If the residents are not bedridden, it is
not unreasonable to ask if there is a bar and adequate privacy. An elegant Boston dowager of some 80 years of age
expressed great concern to me about leaving her home because
she enjoyed two martinis every evening and wanted to have the
privacy to participate in sensual or sexual activity.

Before concluding I would like to stress one fact. The
process of placement is a choosing and without doubt the
most appropriate person to make the choice is the placee, not
the placer. It may not always be possible to abide by the
wishes of the older person, especially if he or she is
suffering some measure of mental impairment. But it is
always our first obligation to honor the elderly individual's choice of where and how to live as much as I would
honor yours and you mine. The tendency to paternalism, no
matter how well meaning, should be avoided.

    The persons placed, and the circumstances of placement,
are not static. Reevaluation must be performed periodically
to assure that the proper level of care yesterday remains
appropriate today. This is true as surely for the patient
who needs services as for the one who requires medicine.
Dosages of both need adjustment over time. Also, consider
that sometimes, for reasons not altogether clear, persons
require fewer services. Diseases may remit, symptoms may
improve, compensatory mechanisms may come into play, requirements may change as may a person's social circumstances.
Nursing homes may then think with increasing interest about
rehabilitation and the stigma attached to these facilities
may fade, if not vanish.

References

(1) Harris, Charles S. Fact Book on Aging: A Profile of
     America's Older Population. Washington, D.C.: National
     Council on the Aging, 1978.
(2) Ibid.
(3) Brody, Elaine. "Aging and Family Personality: A Develop-
     mental View." Family Process 13:23-37, 1974.
(4) Harris. Fact Book on Aging.
(5) Williams, T. Franklin, John G. Hill, Matthew E. Fair-
     banks, and Kenneth G. Knox. "Appropriate Placement
     of the Chronically Ill and Aged, a Successful Approach
     by Evaluation." J.A.M.A. 226:1332-35, 1973.
 6) Ibid.
 7) Steel, K., T. Franklin Williams, M. Fairbanks, and K.
     Knox. "Laboratory Screening in the Evaluation and
     Placement of Geriatric Patients." J. Am. Geriatr.
     Soc. 22:538-43, 1974.
(8) Genesee Region Health Planning Council. Survey of Need
     for Inpatient Beds and Related Home Health Care Ser-
     vices, Monroe County, 1969-70. Rochester, N.Y.:
     Genesee Region Health Planning Council, 1970.
(9) Morton, E. V. and R. M. Tyndall. "Physical Illness in
     Social Emergencies." Gerontological Clinica 13:145-52,
     1971.
(10) Harris. Fact Book on Aging.

Part II

The Health Care System for Elderly Patients

INTRODUCTION

Harold B. Haley

In this section we begin by relating the general systems of
health care for the elderly. Then the home health care
systems and long-term care institutions are described. In
all cases we will be looking at the access to and the operation of the care system.

Frank Mays details some physical and mechanical barriers that make it difficult for elderly patients to receive
the care they need. Also, he presents demographic data
concerning health status of elderly Virginians.

In his second paper, Frank Mays gives a brief statement
of roles of Health Systems Agency in identifying needs of the
elderly and helping develop programs for their care.

From the general access and need problem, Jeanne Miller
gives precise details of what is needed to care for the
elderly patient in the home, including the structure of the
home, the assessment of the patient's status, and housekeeping needs. She explains and gives direction to the family
roles and function in caring for the elderly person at home.
This paper would be of great help to anyone having an elderly
person in their home or to a provider whose patients are
cared for in the home.

Mary Kate House's "how-to" paper is one of two reprinted
from another publication. When we read it, we were struck
by how it personalizes the elements of care detailed by
Jeanne Miller and Mary Lauth.

Mary Elyn Lauth recites the specifics of how a home
health care agency can aid in caring for the elderly by
bringing outside help into the home.

Services given to patients in long-term care facilities
are presented by John Boyd, with emphasis on nursing and
M.D. roles.

Stuart Payne outlines important aspects of the operation
of long-term care facilities and gives examples of problems
in the system relating to Medicare and Medicaid.

CHAPTER 8

SOCIOECONOMIC BARRIERS TO HEALTH CARE

Frank H. Mays

In 1970 about 366,021 Virginians, or 7.9%, were 65 and
older, while eight years later they numbered 463,747, or
9%. This increased longevity emphasizes the need for more
concern about the health problems of the elderly as well as
the logistical problems they encounter in obtaining care
and services. These health and logistical problems, the
progress made, the need to develop plans, and directions
for future care and services will be discussed.

Since 1940 there has been a 3% decrease in death rates
for Virginians (1). There has also been a changing pattern
of mortality and increased longevity at both ends of the
aging spectrum. Under age 15, there has been about a 10%
decrease in death rates since 1940. Deaths age 85 and over
in 1970 represented a 5.8% increase since 1940 (2).

For those retired at age 65 and over, the three greatest causes of death are heart disease, malignant neoplasms,
and cerebrovascular disease (3). Since 1900 there has been
a 5.8% increase in age 65 or older population. Lower birth
rates will further raise this proportion of the elderly. If
the population should grow at the two-child rate, the proportion of age 65 and over would reach 10.6% by the end of the
century. If the two-child average prevailed until the population stabilized, the proportion of the elderly would level
off at about 16%. However, if the population grew at the
three-child rate, in the year 2000 the proportion would be
8.9%, less than it is now.

A study entitled "The Virginia Health Interview Survey,"
recently funded and sponsored by five Virginia Health Systems
Agencies (HSA's) and their counterpart health-planning and
data agencies at state level, is underway and will yield
more precise data on aging and problems of access to care.
However, my conclusions and perceptions about access to
care are divided into these categories:

1. Geographic accessibility to elements of care or
service in space, with consideration of land features such
as topography, terrain, transportation routes, and transportation modes.

2. Temporal accessibility to elements of care or service within certain lengths of time, an important consideration depending on the nature of disease, illness or injury,
and mode of transportation.

3. Financial accessibility to elements of care or service, based on ability to pay or availability of funds from
other than the individual for financing care or services.

Geographic Accessibility

Much of Virginia is rural, with 80% of the population living
in urban land areas. Isolated population clusters containing many elderly persons is a problem in the southwest
Virginia mountains. Major arterial highways and paved
secondary roads are reasonably good, but there are many miles of
circuitous, torturous, two-lane roads. Having to travel
15-20 miles for medical care on some of these roads is a
problem, especially if persons are in pain or fighting for
life. Regardless of locale, geographic access to primary
care for the elderly is a problem. In 1977 the Virginia
Office on Aging stated that "older people have a problem
securing adequate transportation for their personal needs;
while service providers find their budgets must be allocated
to transporting service users to service facilities or for
bringing services to the user" (4).
     Many elderly persons live in areas with inadequate or
no public transportation system and rely on private automobiles. Automobile costs and sometimes physical problems
make many elderly persons dependent on friends, relatives,
or volunteers for transportation.
     Elderly residents of rural areas face special problems.
Low incomes hinder car ownership and maintenance. In addition, neighbors may be several miles away, roads may be
poor, and distances to essential services may be great,
making securing transportation more difficult. Distance
between elderly residents makes it costly for service providers, who wish to provide door-to-door rides related to
offered services. With few exceptions, rural areas have
little or no bus service.
     Numerous programs could benefit the elderly in need of
service-related transportation. However, there are some
problems. Many of these potential resources are used to
serve all age groups. For a variety of reasons, elderly
persons require some special provisions that cannot be
accommodated without some specific funding sources. Secondly, the funding sources favor expenditures for equipment,
either by laws establishing the funds (Urban Mass Transit
Authority 16b[2] program) or by the short-term anticipated
life span of the resource. Sources of funds for operating
transportation services (drivers, fuel, maintenance) are
more limited. Further, various restrictions placed on each
funding stream make coordination most difficult.
     The final and most discouraging characteristic of
transportation to services is the state of the art itself.
Despite recognition of the importance of transportation,
despite resources available to address certain needs, and
despite a large number of model projects across the country,
there is no agreement on the most efficient and appropriate
transportation system. The result is that there is no

system but rather a series of piecemeal efforts made at a
sometimes staggering cost.

Elderly persons have special transportation problems.
Some need escorts, some need special physical accommodation,
some could benefit from mass transit not now available, and
many simply need income or subsidies to buy services.

Public monies are, or could be, used in providing transportation for older persons. Some funds are administered
directly by federal agencies such as ACTION, while most are
administered by state or local agencies using federal funds.
Each funding source has its own restrictions, eligibility
criteria, application procedures, funding period, and coverage area. For example, in Virginia, Title III Older Americans Act monies used for transportation are administered
by the Office on Aging at the state level and by Area Agencies on Aging at the local level. Eligible riders include
anyone age 60 and over. Title XX of the Social Security
Act is administered by two state-level agencies, the Department of Welfare and the Commission for the Visually Handicapped, and its funds are allocated to forty-three local
welfare departments for their use. Eligible recipients of
Title XX funded transportation must meet income requirements
established at the state level. Urban Mass Transit Authority monies are administered by the State Department of Highways and Transportation and awarded only to local nonprofit
agencies. Eligible riders include the elderly and the handicapped. There is an obvious problem for localities wishing
to provide a comprehensive and coordinated transportation
service using these varied resources.

In addition to individual grant programs, there are
several local attempts to integrate funding streams, including the Roanoke RADAR Program, JAUNT in the Charlottesville
area, and CORDET in the Richmond area, representing combined efforts of a variety of social service agencies to
use pooled transportation resources. The approach is to
centralize equipment, maintenance, drivers, and dispatching
and thereby produce cost savings. These programs are in
early stages of development or operation, and evaluation
is not yet possible or appropriate. Spearheaded by the
Tidewater Area Agencies on Aging serving some 25 to 30
jurisdictions, transportation of elderly persons depends
upon their ability to pay fares, to safely board a vehicle,
to walk to and from bus stops, and availability of escorts
when needed   Transit operators who receive federal funds
are required to provide reduced fare rates, usually one-half
the normal rate, to elderly persons riding in off-peak hours.

Many elderly persons rely on their private automobiles.
Their activities as drivers and pedestrians have been of
concern to state and local legislators and planners. Virginia, unlike many other states, does not have special
requirements for the elderly who seek to obtain or renew

drivers licenses. Studies (5) on the value of these requirements, reaction time of older drivers, accident rates for
older drivers and pedestrians, and related topics show:
     1. Chronological age is only a rough, and sometimes
inaccurate, indicator of the capacity of older drivers.
While aging itself is associated with deteriorating vision
and hearing, relationship between specific problems and
driving performance is not clear and at least one expert
feels that drivers should be examined individually, rather
than as an age group.
     2. Older drivers do have higher accident rates than
drivers in their middle years, but because they drive less,
their total number of accidents is not as great as other
age groups. The aging driver tends to be involved in less
serious accidents, with a lower incidence of excessive speed
or drinking.
     3. Some elderly are at a disadvantage when driving
because they learned to drive when the highway system was
less complex, they lack knowledge about safe driving skills,
they may not be informed about effects of medication on
driving performance, and traffic signs and signals do not
take into account problems related to possible deficiencies
in visual discrimination, short-term memory, and logical
interpretation of stimuli.
     4. Elderly persons do less driving during rush hours,
night hours, the winter, and difficult daily driving situations.
     Research seems to indicate that the elderly do have
higher accident rates as drivers for a variety of reasons
not always directly associated with chronological age, but
as a group, they drive fewer miles than younger drivers
and they exercise caution in driving habits and in avoidance
of hazardous driving situations. Therefore, the actual
number of accidents in which they are involved is not high.
     According to the National Safety Council (6), 12% of
all motor vehicle fatalities (5,780 in 1975) were persons
age 65 or over, as follows: killed in collisions, 2,600;
killed in noncollisions, 750; as pedestrians, 2,110; in
collisions with a fixed object, 170; in collisions with a
train, 120; in collisions with a pedal cycle, 30.
     In Virginia there are 221,598 licensed drivers over
age 65. In 1975 Virginia State Police indicated that 8,461
drivers age 65 or over were involved in auto accidents. Of
1,030 total deaths due to auto accidents, 117, or 11.4%,
were age 65 or over. A serious concern, both in state and
national statistics, is the pedestrian death rate. Nationally, 25% of all motor-vehicle-related deaths of older persons were pedestrian deaths, while in Virginia in 1975 there
were 36.8%, or a total of 43 older pedestrian deaths. The
elderly are overrepresented in traffic fatalities involving
pedestrians (7).

In obtaining geographic access to care or service for
elderly, transportation is essential. In 1976 surveys of
area agencies on aging, three types of services were identified where transportation was most in need: health services, shopping, and senior activity center functions (8).

Temporal Accessibility

The length of time required to obtain care or services is a
major consideration when considering access to care for the
elderly.
     Access to primary medical and dental care for some 12
to 15 population clusters of 2,500 or more persons in southwest Virginia often exceeds the standard 30-45 minute drive
accepted by medical professionals and communities. Many
emergency conditions exist where medical care is mandatory
within 5-10 minutes in order to reverse a traumatic episode.
Many die, including the elderly, when an acute episode could
have been reversed if definitive care were provided in time.
If the situation is life threatening, definitive care will
begin immediately once the individual is in the hands of
medical professionals.
     Improving response times for emergency medical services
are now beginning in southwest Virginia and across the state.
There is more in-depth training of emergency medical techni-
cians and emergency department personnel, more sophisticated
radio communication systems between prehospital emergency
services and hospital emergency departments, more self-help
training of citizens in greater volume who can respond to
potential drownings, cardiac arrests, and other life-threatening episodes.
     Forty-five minutes to one hour waiting time in a doc-
tor's office can be a problem for elderly persons. Some
professionals recognize this problem, but there are emer-
gencies to deal with as well as scheduled appointments. A
stress situation is sometimes created when waiting time
at the doctor's office exceeds 45 minutes to one hour, because volunteer drivers cannot fulfill other commitments
later on in the day. The elderly person sometimes finds the
volunteer driver less willing to provide transportation for
the next doctor's appointment.

Financial Accessibility

According to the Virginia Office on Aging, 30% of Virginia's
elderly have less than poverty-level incomes. Last year
this income was $5,750 for a nonfarm family of four with a
male head of household (9). Need for adequate income is
related to every other need faced by older citizens. Rising
food, housing, health, and transportation costs are devastating to the elderly, who are disproportionately poor,
heavily reliant on fixed or limited income sources, such as

Social Security, and not likely to be in the labor force. Many older persons have retired or have been retired involuntarily due to their disabilities and find their savings and their pensions decimated by rising costs of essential goods and services.

Although some retired older persons have earnings, annuities, and other income-producing assets, Social Security is their major source of income. About five-sixths of the older population rely on Social Security checks for the major part of their income. Average payments from Social Security in 1979 were: single men $292 per month; widows, $265 per month; and disabled, $320 per month (10). Social Security and other retirement income programs increase the above-average income for some, but not the majority. There are Supplemental Security Income (SSI), private pensions, Veteran's Pensions, Railroad Retirement, Civil Service Retirement, and Virginia Supplemental Retirement.

Health services for elderly range from ambulatory, acute, nursing home, long-term institutionalization to residential care. These services are expensive because the elderly use such services more often than other age groups. Payments for such services come from tax dollars paid into the Social Security System over the years by the labor force or into general and special funds of state treasuries. The Virginia Office on Aging Plan states that it costs about $12,000 per year for one person's stay in a skilled nursing home, about $9,000 per year in an intermediate care nursing home, and $8,820 per year for hospitalization in a state mental health institution (11).

For acute hospital and medical care, Medicare is the primary payment source for many persons over age 65. Social Security officials state that medicare pays only 34%-40% of total costs for health and medical care of the aging. Are these costs being written off as uncollectible by health institutions and professionals, or are these costs being paid by the elderly?

Also, many elderly benefit from the Medicaid program designed to benefit those who are disabled and needy under statutes such as Aid to Permanently and Totally Disabled, Aid to the Blind, and the like. In addition, about 75% of persons age 65 and over carry some private health insurance that pays only 5.2% of their health care expenses.

Overall, financial resources to provide access to care are available, except for physical exams, dental care, non-prescription drugs, personal comfort items, eyeglasses, and hearing aids.

However, an unknown amount of out-of-pocket payments are made for items that enhance the health and well-being of the elderly. In the future we should consider defraying these extra costs so that the elderly will have fewer costs to contend with in maintaining their health.

    In summary, we must be flexible in dealing with the
needs and problems of the elderly. The elderly have participated in the labor force and affairs which have shaped
this nation and have benefited the younger generation by
their presence and knowledge. Improving access to care in
all respects must be of paramount concern. We must all
respect our elders and demonstrate sincere human warmth
for them individually and collectively.

References

 (1) Virginia Department of Health. Statistical Annual
      Report . Richmond: Virginia Department of Health, 1975,
      p. 10.
 (2) Ibid., p. 26.
 (3) Ibid., p. 28.
 (4) Virginia Office on Aging. Virginia's Direction in
      Aging: A Timely Matter. Richmond: Virginia Office
      on Aging, February 1, 1977, p. 68.
 (5) Ibid., pp. 77-78.
 (6) Ibid., p. 78.
 (7) Ibid.
 (8) Ibid., p. 69.
 (9) Ibid., p. 41.
(10) Ibid., p. 42.
(11) Ibid., pp. 51-54.

CHAPTER 9

HEALTH SYSTEMS AGENCIES IN THE CARE OF THE AGED

Frank H. Mays

Represented in most areas of this country today are organizations called Health Systems Agencies (HSA). Our function
is health-system planning, project review, and being an
agent for research and development. The HSA is mainly supported by federal grants, although we are organized as a
voluntary, nonstock, not-for-profit corporation. HSA's
cover the country. This presentation shows the involvement
of one HSA in health problems of the aged.

Our mission is to describe and document all facets of
the health care system and to make recommendations for future
directions in health-system development through a published
Health Systems Plan. Our HSA covers one-third of Virginia,
about 13,000 square miles, and serves about 1,100,000 persons.
In southwest Virginia we encounter many health-related resources. For example, our service covers eight public health
districts; eight community mental health, mental retardation,
and substance-abuse service boards; several medical and dental societies; more than three dozen short-stay community
hospitals; some forty nursing homes; a University of Virginia
School of Medicine second facility in the Roanoke-Lynchburg
area; seven area agencies on aging; one Veterans Administration Medical Center; three state mental hospitals; and two
mental retardation training centers and hospitals.

The HSA Board of Directors is a cross-section of health
care professionals and citizens. The board structure gives
majority representation to consumers, those who derive no
income from providing health services. This structure
provides a more objective viewpoint for the plans and recommendations made for improving health status and health systems and a more coordinated process than if each professional organization functioned separately.

In planning a health care system for the future, we
found deficiencies and excesses in the present health
system which needed to be corrected if our citizens, and
especially our elderly, are to receive maximum benefit. Our
service is not a "hands-on" kind of service which provides
directly for the needs of the elderly, but rather a service
that identifies service needs through planning. Some service
needs are:
     1. The elderly need a system of care that provides
prompt accessibility to acute episodic care and emergency
care. Many acute episodes, such as cardiac arrests,
respiratory infections, accidents, and burns might be
reversible if definitive care and treatment could be provided quickly. The emergency care system needs development,
and we will continue to work for this further development.

2. In this health service area, there are a dozen
isolated population groups of 2,500 or more persons where
the provision of primary, front-line medical and dental care
is inadequate. We will continue to work with these areas
and with organizations such as the Virginia Council on
Health and Medical Care, National Health Service Corps,
and others to develop the necessary resources.

3. Essential services need to be convenient for the
elderly. The elderly have to move from place to place
during one episode of obtaining medical care, and in some of
our areas, helping agencies should try getting together to
provide "one-stop" services.

4. Obtaining transportation is a major problem for
the elderly. There seems to be no simple solution, but we
will continue to address this transportation problem in our
planning activities.

5. Accessibility to home health care provided by medical, nursing, and allied health professionals is a significant need, and this kind of care is neither fully developed
nor accepted by third-party payers and medical professionals.
Contrary to the belief that home health care will be costly
and less effective, we know the New River Valley Agency on
Aging provides homemaker and health-related services for
$6.90 per hour. A hospital recently reported $5.60 per hour
for providing hospital care, with an average patient day
cost of $134.40. Home health care can be definitive and
effective care with adequate support and supervision by
physicians, and there would be fewer hours of individualized
patient care to which cost could be assigned.

6. The HSA is constantly trying to improve and add to
its data base so that rational decisions can be made. We
are cosponsoring a statewide health interview survey that
will provide us with more information about the health status
of certain age groups in the population, utilization of services, and problems encountered in obtaining services.

7. An interdisciplinary communications linkage must
be established.

CHAPTER 10

THE FAMILY AND THE CARE OF THE ELDERLY PERSON AT HOME

Jeanne C. Miller

Many older persons prefer to stay in their homes rather than
move to protective residences or nursing homes. Care of
these persons and relationships with their families require
consideration of many factors.

Home Environment

The home environment of the elderly should be explored.
Usually, the home environment contributes to our physical,
social, and psychological well-being. Because of increasing
time spent in the home during later life, this environment
is important as a source of contentment or a source of stress.
     The home environment should be both safe and pleasant.
Some characteristics identified by numerous authors as contributing to home safety for older persons are:
     1. A residence with low maintenance--permanent storm
windows and screens, central air and heat.
     2. Adequate lighting, including night lights and a
flashlight beside the older person's bed and well-lighted
stairways.
     3. Absence of loose extension cords, small mats, slid-
ing rugs or rugs with high edges, slippery hardwood or lino-
leum floors.
     4. Handrails in good repair in hallways, on staircases,
and in bathrooms beside commodes and in and around showers.
     5. Telephone in living room or kitchen plus at bed-
side with dials in large print and a list of emergency and
most frequently called numbers in large print at both
locations.
     6. Absence of small tables or stools, sharp cornered
or rickety furniture--rooms free of clutter.
     7. One-floor residence, if possible, without stairs.
However, if not possible, top and bottom steps should be
accented (painted white).
     8. Well-lighted, well-labeled medicine area.
     9. An electric stove, if possible, with large distinct
markings to indicate heat level and on and off positions.
     10. A kitchen designed for easy movement--big enough
for a wheel chair. Sinks, other appliances (i.e., oven,
refrigerator) and cabinets placed at a level to discourage
bending and possible dizziness.
     11. A high toilet with handrails.
     12. Nonskid surface in shower--shower preferred over
tub--controls outside shower or tub.
     13. Adequate locks that can be operated by resident.

14. Ramps--nonslippery--to house entrance.
Safety precautions of the elderly at home include:
1. Avoid bending to avoid dizziness--get up slowly.
2. Arrange for someone to do maintenance work (clear
snow, mow grass, change storm windows, etc.).
3. Avoid looking up when climbing stairs or suddenly
moving head from side to side.
4. If taking medications, keep a simple, clear medicine
chart that includes: name of medication, time due, and a
place to check off when the medication is actually taken.
5. Always take the time to turn on lights rather than
risk falling over something in the dark.
6. Don't rush or panic.
7. If weakness while showering is a problem, use a
nonskid slatted bench for sitting, rather than risk falling
while getting in and out of the tub.
8. Avoid furniture rearrangements as they may cause
confusion.
While the above factors contribute to a safe home
environment, other factors contributing to pleasurable
surroundings include:
1. Familiar items in familiar places: photographs and
paintings, furniture, plants, radio and/or television.
2. Brighter wall colors than in younger days due to
decreasing eyesight; however, possibility of sun glare must
be considered.
3. Windows for sunlight.
4. A sitting room with comfortable chairs for visitors.
5. Clocks, calendars, and mirrors in accessible locations.

General Assessment of the Older Person at Home

In addition to assessing the safety and comfort of an older
person's home, it is important to determine the individual's
functional status so that appropriate assistance can be provided. The purpose of such an assessment is not to focus
on weaknesses but to determine how the patient can best be
maintained at a high level of functioning. This requires
focusing on client assets as well as disabilities and allows
the nurse to assist the family in identifying what should
not be done for the older member as well as determining the
most appropriate assistance for specific problems.
Many investigators and practitioners have developed
assessment tools helpful in working with older clients. The
functioning assessed by most of these tools includes: daily
personal care, mobility, general health status, usual housekeeping, ability to provide food for self, budget skills and
financial resources, social participation, and cognition-
mental status.
In assessing an individual's ability to care for himself, it is important to determine whether he can get in

and out of the bed without assistance, get on and off the toilet, in and out of the bath, dress and groom self (shave, comb hair, care for teeth and nails), and put on, adjust, and maintain devices such as hearing aids. Assess mobility by determining whether an individual can get in and out of bed without difficulty, walk around the room, climb and descend stairs, walk a block, swim or jog or participate in active sports, drive a car, get around the community via public transportation, and travel long distances.

Factors to consider in evaluating general health status include: does the client regularly see a family physician? When was he/she last seen? Is dizziness, unsteadiness, or fainting a problem? Does the client regularly have teeth, hearing, and eyesight evaluated and are there working corrective devices? Are there particular problems with eating, urination, or bowel movements? What chronic conditions does the patient report? Are medications safely stored and correctly taken?

Housekeeping abilities need to be assessed only if the client has no one to regularly provide these services. However, a client's involvement in these daily chores may significantly contribute to his feelings of self-worth and independence, and, therefore, should be encouraged.

Assessing housekeeping functioning includes evaluating the individual's ability to dust furniture, vacuum, do laundry, wash dishes, keep appliances and cupboards clean, work in the yard, and provide usual house maintenance. Also, we need to evaluate the individual's ability to buy and prepare nutritious food, including "special diets."

Often overlooked is the individual's ability to manage household accounts and financial affairs. Can and does the individual pay bills, write checks, keep a record of income and expenditures, manage own income or have a financial advisor who monitors and controls client's investments and income?

Assess the older person's pattern of social activity and compare with prior patterns of activity. Does the individual have family and friends with whom he has contact on a regular basis at least twice a week? Does the individual have someone identified to call in an emergency? Does the individual regularly attend day care, senior center, club meetings, church? If the individual attends any of the above, with what frequency does he/she attend? Is the individual satisfied with his level of social activity?

Finally, because of the possibility of cognition problems, the individual's mental status needs to be evaluated. There are many forms of mental status examinations available. Goldfarb's (1973) Mental Status Examination is frequently utilized and includes the following items:

Where are we now?

Where is this place (located)?

What is today's date (day or month)?
What month is it?
What year is it?
How old are you?
What is your birthday?
What year were you born?
Who is the president of the United States?
Who was the president before him?

Two or less errors on the above test indicate that the problems in cognition are probably absent or mild. Three through eight errors suggest moderate dysfunction, while nine to ten errors suggest severe dysfunction.

This assessment is superficial and does not replace a thorough physical and social-psychological examination needed by all elderly persons at regular intervals. However, the above assessment allows identification of the individual's ability to manage daily affairs and determines areas of functioning that need to be supported by family or other caring persons.

The nurse or health worker providing this assessment should teach family or other caring persons about the process. Then they could utilize these tools to evaluate changes in functioning of older persons and modify their assistance of these older persons.

Assisting Families and Elderly Depressed Members at Home

Despite attention to the above factors, there are older persons who develop psychological or emotional difficulties who choose to live at home. Special problems arise with families or other caring persons who are attempting to maintain the older person with such difficulties who lives in the community. Professionals working in the field of aging should provide information for the elderly and their families that will assist them in understanding and coping with these psychological difficulties.

There is a need for more mental health service for the elderly in the community. However, few mental health services are directed toward supporting the elderly in their homes.

In outlining a proposed plan for comprehensive mental health service for the elderly, the Task Force on Mental Health Needs of the Elderly in Virginia recommended that:

1. All elderly persons be provided the services of advocacy and public education.

2. Older persons suspected of being mentally ill should be provided multiphasic screening and case management services.

3. The at-risk elderly populations should be provided telephone/visitor contact services, social centers, and alternate housing; the mentally ill elderly should be

provided emergency outpatient, partial hospitalization, inpatient, day care, and alternate housing services.

4. Former mental patients who are elderly should be
provided follow-up services, therapeutic activities centers,
day care services, and alternate housing.

5. Agencies and agents providing services to the
elderly should be provided consultation and specialized
training concerned with mental health of the elderly.

One priority underlying this comprehensive plan is prevention of emotional or mental disability of elderly persons
in their homes and assistance of older persons living at home
with such disabilities. Assistance includes both direct care
of such a patient and support of others providing such care.

Depression is the most frequently occurring and least
recognized emotional difficulty experienced by the elderly.
Families and elderly persons do not think about the multiple, cumulative losses which older people regularly experience or the probable effects of these losses on the individual's emotional state. Older individuals and their families
should be informed about depression, preferably prior to
experiencing these losses. This suggests the need for preventive intervention during preretirement years.

Some helpful information about depression for the
elderly and their families is presented below. The simplis-
tic nature of this presentation is recognized.

First, depression is generally related to an individual's reaction to losses. Older people experience many of
the following losses: loss of occupational position, loss
of position of power in the family, loss of friends, siblings,
spouses, loss of physical strength and agility, loss of
mobility, and loss of independence.

Common symptoms of depression include: feelings of
listlessness, poor appetite, declining interest in the world
in general, difficulty sleeping, early morning wakefulness,
overconcern with body, inactivity, lack of expressiveness,
and overwhelming feelings of sadness. Generally, when people experience depression they withdraw from social relationships and normal activities. Increasing isolation tends to
lead to increasing suspiciousness. One outcome of this
spiraling process is the family's perception of the depressed older person as senile.

Some guidelines for assisting families maintaining an
older depressed member in the community include:

1. Help the family accept and discuss its own frus-
trations in dealing with older member.

2. Help the family identify and recognize perceived
losses that the older member has experienced.

3. Assist the family in encouraging the older member
to talk about his/her perceived losses and experiences with
aging.

4. Encourage the family to actively work at maintaining

the older depressed member's involvement with other people
and a meaningful daily routine.

5. Inform family members of programs for the elderly
in the community (Senior Centers, Gray Panthers, RSVP) and
facilitate client's relationship with these programs.

6. Discuss with the family the basic human need for
recognition and involvement with others. Older people who
believe that they are needed by someone are not as likely to
be depressed.

7. Discuss research findings on well-being in older
persons with the family, for example, staying in training--
intellectually, socially, and physically--is positively
correlated with general good health in the elderly.

8. Suggest that the family arrange for client to have
a thorough physical examination if this has not been done
recently.

9. Discuss with the family the usual processes involved
in depression and the pathological, debilitating functions
depression can serve for the individual. Depression is frequently the result of feeling let down or disappointed and
leads to anger that changes to guilt. Unfortunately, depression is not easily self-controlled and it does sometimes
allow clients to control families and others, permits the
client to avoid interactions and responsibilities, and it
is often an attempt to satisfy dependency needs.

10. Discuss with the family the need to be aware of a
suicide risk and help them recognize when a family member
should receive professional intervention. Point out clues
to suicide such as: the individual puts affairs in order,
gives away possessions, suddenly appears calm, relieved,
less depressed, talks about ending it all, going on a trip,
seeing a dead friend or relative, and collects means for
attempting suicide (pills, gun).

11. Families need to be informed that sometimes it is
necessary to provide medication for depressed persons. Frequently, antidepressants should not be used in combination
with other drugs. Families need to know that they can
call on psychiatrists to evaluate the need for, and appropriateness of, medications for older depressed family
members.

Health workers should assist families to recognize that
a withdrawn, seemingly senile, older person may simply be
overwhelmed by depression. Appropriate intervention by the
family can result in a radical change in the client's
behavior.

Memory Loss and Memory Disturbance

Memory loss and memory disturbance are problems frequently
identified as characteristics of old age. However, there is
little evidence that most older persons do have serious

memory disturbances. Studies show that older persons themselves who complain of memory loss do not generally demonstrate functional evidence of this loss. In fact, it is more
common that the individual who complains of poor memory
actually is depressed and the complaint is related to low
self-esteem (Epstein 1976). Usually memory losses or memory
changes are reported by spouses, friends, or other family
members. The impaired patient is usually unconcerned.

Many persons who have been diagnosed as suffering from
senile dementia actually have demonstrated symptoms caused
by sensory deficits (i.e., hearing and sight loss) and
social isolation. Health workers need to carefully assess
clients who have been, or may be, labeled as having organic
brain syndrome for confounding losses, physical and social
problems.

There are older persons who exhibit symptoms of memory
disturbance. Families attempting to maintain older members
in the community need to understand something about these
disturbances and interventions with confused older persons.
The following discussion has been developed for the elderly
and their families.

Mental confusion may be experienced by anyone at any
age as a result of many different factors. However, recurring mental confusion unrelated to high fever, extreme
physical or emotional stress, or toxins is more common among
the elderly.

In some older people a condition develops which includes
the following symptoms: memory disturbance or impairment,
impaired intellectual functioning, impaired judgment, impaired orientation to people, places, things, and changeable
or inappropriate moods or affect. These symptoms range in
severity from slight (which causes little interference with
everyday life) to severe (which makes it impossible for the
individual to function outside a protected environment).
Symptoms may be reversible, such as when an individual
develops the above symptoms with a physical illness or a
fever. Symptoms may also be permanent as in chronic brain
disorder.

There are two major types of chronic brain syndrome.
However, this disorder is referred to as senility with senile
psychosis. There is progressive decline in memory and
intellectual function and judgment. The individual may
appear apathetic (unfeeling) and tends to become more and
more confused, with rambling speech and suspicious tenden-
cies. The second type of chronic brain syndrome is caused
by arteriosclerosis (hardening of the arteries). With this
disorder, progression is uneven compared with a steady
decline of senile psychosis. Early symptoms include:
dizziness, headaches, decreased mental and physical vigor,
gradual intellectual loss, and spotty memory impairment.

Acute brain syndrome, or reversible brain disorder, is characterized by a fluctuating level of awareness, hallucinations (seeing or hearing things that aren't there), mistaking one person for another, restlessness, anxiety, and lack of cooperativeness. Some causes of acute brain syndrome include congestive heart failure, malnutrition, infection, strokes, drugs (diuretics, steroids, barbiturates, tranquilizers, inomethacin, L-Dopa), head injury, alcohol, diabetes, liver failure and dehydration.

If an older person develops the above symptoms, it is important that families contact a physician. The physician should be informed of all medications taken by the client (including laxatives, cold medicines, aspirin, nonprescription or sleeping pills).

While chronic brain syndrome can be overwhelming to family members, some interventions which can be helpful include making lists, keeping things in obvious places for the older person, arranging with someone to check on the client to make sure the client eats regularly, and to remind the older person of appointments, arrange for the client to read the newspaper and talk about what's happening in the world, maintain a daily schedule--keep it posted on a bulletin board beside a clock if necessary--keep things as consistent as possible for the older confused person. Don't panic when you find the older person very confused. Instead, slowly and consistently reinforce reality, and be certain the older person carries adequate identification when going out (an identification bracelet which cannot be removed is useful), and evaluate the safety of the client's home.

The information on sensory deprivation is helpful when considering interventions with acute brain syndrome. Keep some familiar things around, keep a watch and radio nearby, and encourage the older person to use these; don't allow the patient to withdraw because he is confused, but encourage him to talk to people about his experience; tell the patient what time it is, what day it is and what you will be doing during the day; keep telling him where he is and what is being done; visit him frequently. Don't tell him to "just rest" when he asks questions as this tends to increase anxiety; answer questions simply--long explanations may be confusing.

Just because an older person may be forgetful and can't think as fast and as clearly as he did in the past, it does not mean that he will need to be institutionalized. Remind the confused older person that each person who may periodically experience confusion can help himself through accepting that not all forgetfulness is progressive, keeping his mind active, reading, discussing and thinking about things which interests him, simplifying and organizing daily life with checklists in obvious places, maintaining a daily routine,

and asking someone to check on him and help him out from
time to time.

Finally, families need to remember that increasing
isolation may cause older persons to develop symptoms similar to senile dementia. It also is not uncommon for older
people who aren't generally confused to be confused in
stressful, emotional, and physical situations. For instance,
an anniversary of a death of someone close, a trip, a change
of residence, hospitalization, redecoration or renovation
of a home may all precipitate an episode of confusion.

Families can be most helpful by being consistent, maintaining a regular schedule of visits, decreasing the uncer-
tainty experienced by the older person so he can predict
what will happen and experience a sense of control, and
communicating in clear simple language. Furthermore, families must be aware of the need for regular assessment of the
older person's hearing and sight to decrease the risk of
unnecessary isolation and confusion.

Interpersonal Difficulties of Older Persons at Home

While it is common knowledge that human beings experience
both gratification and suffering as a result of interpersonal relationships, somehow we expect older persons to have
no interpersonal problems. This is unrealistic. Families
with older members need to be aware of common interpersonal
difficulties experienced by the elderly. The following
information is presented for them.

Older people frequently experience interpersonal
problems with spouses. These may take many forms and be
precipitated by many different events. A major event which
greatly affects the elderly is retirement. If a husband
has worked and the wife remained at home, both spouses may
have a difficult time coping with the change in their routine, their increased contacts with each other, and the way
their friendships with others are affected by this change of
status.

Frequently, much of a couple's social life revolves
around work acquaintances. Retirement leads to a decrease
in invitations and a decline in social activity. Both
spouses may feel rejected and handle this loss in a variety
of ways: blame each other for the loss; withdraw from other
social relationships and become increasingly dependent on
each other; make increased demands on family members for
social interaction; renew old friendships which have not
been cultivated for many years; or strike out in search of
new activities and friendships--social clubs, senior citizen
centers, volunteer work, new or expanding hobbies, or new
work.

The losses associated with retirement may be difficult
to accept. However, more satisfactory personal relationships may develop after retirement because people have the

time to invest in friendship. The following suggestions
are made for assisting elderly persons coping with the
problems of retirement related to marital relationships.
First, encourage older persons to discuss these changes with
their spouses, keep the communication channels open to prevent the development of long-term resentment and unhappiness.
Secondly, retirement also means that most couples spend more
time together than they ever have before. A wife may feel
that her husband is in the way and resent his interference
with her daily schedule. He may feel unneeded. Encourage
both spouses to compromise. Both routines must change to
accommodate changing needs. Finally, it is not uncommon
that a husband and wife may both work and the husband's
retirement may precede his wife's by several years. Unless
part-time work, hobbies, or adjustments in household routines
have been arranged, the husband may experience an overwhelming sense of uselessness. Once again, discussing this openly
is crucial for successful adaptation.

Many older people express a sense of loss of contact
with other human beings. Human touch is very important in
normal development. Infants need human touch to thrive.
As children we all touch and are touched with loving caresses
by many people (parents, grandparents, other children, aunts
and uncles). As adolescents and then as young married
couples, we explore touch as a form of communication. When
we become parents we set the stage for many years of hugs,
pats, and pokes. But, as children grow up and we grow older,
the touching decreases drastically.

Some people have attempted to artifically establish a
sense of love based on touching through such methods as
sensitivity training. Relationships based on a natural
sense of caring may be more satisfying than those developed
through such contrived experiences. However, such training
may reawaken a sense of pleasure experienced through close
relationships. This reawakening may motivate older persons
to establish new close and meaningful relationships. Anyone
planning to become involved in such a group should carefully
determine the training and skill of the leader prior to
participation.

Numerous voluntary activities provide the opportunity
for loving relationships with other human beings. Some of
these are: volunteer work in hospitals, visiting homefast
elderly people--writing letters, performing small tasks--
foster grandparents' organizations, helping with the nur-
sery during church services so young mothers can have a
quiet hour away from children, teaching Bible school, and
serving as a teacher's aide one day a week. In addition,
if grandparents live close enough to children, it may be
feasible to have them baby-sit for short periods on a
regular basis.

Unfortunately, death is a part of interpersonal

relationships. For the older person it is a reality which
is faced repeatedly. Loss of lifetime friends, spouses, or
children are all difficult to accept. Coping with death
varies from one individual to another. However, some common
behaviors associated with normal grief include: shock,
horror, denial or relief at the news of the death, crying,
remembering, feeling lost and abandoned, going through the
motions of life feeling empty, gradual resumption of activity, and continuation of life without the dead person. Normally, this process can involve as much as a year to complete.

Sometimes people experience an abnormal grief reaction,
the most common of which is delayed grief. In this case,
the individual is unable to mourn (can't cry, can't talk
about it, simply can't accept the death). Generally these
people will insist on leaving clothing, houses, and estates
just as they were prior to the individual's death. Eventually, these persons frequently develop numerous physical
symptoms. They complain of night sweats and nightmares.
They feel they are visited by the deceased in their sleep.

Such abnormal grieving requires the help of a counselor. The condition can be successfully treated, so the
individual is able to grieve and return to normal functioning. Exaggerated grief also occurs in which a serious
depression develops from the experience of loss. Once
again, professional treatment is advisable.

Coping with death is difficult at any age, but particularly for the elderly because of their realization that they
too will die in the not so distant future. Talking about
these thoughts with friends, family, and minister may be
useful in developing satisfactory methods of coping. Many
elderly people have said that experience with death causes
them to feel a sense of urgency about sharing what one knows
and can do with younger people. Through sharing, something
of one's self can live on. When an older person loses a
child, sometimes he/she experiences a sense of guilt--wondering
why he/she continues to live. Such guilt is not realistic
and can best be coped with through renewed efforts to encourage the elderly to share themselves with others through
volunteer activities or other social involvements.

Illness frequently affects interpersonal relationships
between spouses and other family members. Initially, people
want to help. They are concerned and they care. Unfortunately, chronic illness is common in old age and may
severely strain relationships within a family.

As an illness wears on, the well spouse and other family
members (if they are involved) are likely to feel overburdened and trapped. The physical effort required to care for
someone who is debilitated is exhausting. Frequently, the
financial burden of illness is overwhelming. The well spouse
or family members have little free time and, generally, must
put aside their own needs for attention and love to meet

the needs of the ill member. Resentment builds and with
this comes guilt. The ill individual senses the resentment
and feels rejected and defeated. Frequently, he/she is
envious of the well family member's ability to get around.
Furthermore, because dependence and helplessness are very
difficult to accept, the ill member may feel that the family
wishes him/her dead and that they are not providing enough
care. Obviously, these feelings of both the sick and the
well family members result in an increase in tension.

If at all possible, it is most helpful to have some
outsider share the responsibility for the sick member so
that no one person is always responsible (home health aides,
visiting nurses, etc.). Furthermore, arranging a schedule
which is agreeable to both the sick and well family members
decreases expectations and uncertainties which lead to
frustration and guilt.

Discussing feelings as they arise, accepting them as
normal, and trying to work out ways of coping frequently
relieve pent-up anger.

Finally, family members should not give up all to care
for a sick family member. If family members are exhausted,
have no social contacts, and receive no gratification, they
will not be able to effectively care for the sick person.
Family members should not be afraid to ask for help.

Interpersonal relationships between elderly parents
and their children are generally both gratifying and
problematic. Both aspects are unavoidable. Most parents
want to see their children succeed, and indeed, share pleasure and pride in their success. However, parents also
frequently feel left out of the child's success and they
may feel the grown child does not express enough gratitude
for their contribution to his/her success.

Growing up and growing old are both processes of
differentiation. Differentiation means developing a sense
of self: a clear idea of who one is, what one's values are,
and what one will do and will not do. Because of this
differentiation process, there are bound to be differences
between adult children and their parents in some areas.
If all elderly people and all adult children were one hundred
percent mature or differentiated, these differences in values,
mores, beliefs, and behaviors would simply be stated but
would not cause feelings of anger, rejection, guilt, and
disappointment. However, most humans aren't that mature,
so differences are likely to lead to the above feelings.
Such feelings are frequently the reason adult children
see their aging parents so infrequently. They may feel
that their parents are demanding and interfering. Elderly
parents may see their children as ungrateful, rejecting,
and uncaring.

It is difficult for parents to let go of their children
as children and begin to relate to them as grown people. At

the same time, grown children struggle to not respond as
"father's little girl" or "mother's little boy." Furthermore, grown children continue to expect parents to approve
of their behavior and they are uncomfortable when aged parents ask for their support as a friend. Common areas of
interpersonal difficulties between aged persons and their
children include: frequency of visiting (the most common
problem), occasional financial support of the aged parents,
although most aged parents ask for very little in this regard,
decisions about where aged parents will live when they are no
longer able to maintain the "family residence," and grand-
children's behavior and adult children's management of this.
Both parties in the above conflicts must learn to respect
each other as they would respect friends or colleagues. It
is important to recognize and accept that disagreement does
not mean rejection of the individual. If parents and children can be straightforward about their needs, expectations,
and capacities, relationships are likely to be less stressful and more satisfying for both parties. Where possible,
each person must be responsible for his part in the relationship.
     If tension builds in the family, discussing the problem
with a friend or confidant to get an objective opinion may
be helpful before discussing things openly in the family.
Tiptoeing around a problem never makes it go away. Family
members, who automatically make decisions for elderly family
members, do not contribute to the well-being of the elderly.
Every person needs to feel a sense of self-control which
comes through making decisions and sharing decision making.
     Nurses working with families caring for elderly members
in their home must be aware of the multiple interpersonal
stresses experienced by both the older individual and the
family. Encouraging families and clients to discuss these
difficulties and seek appropriate professional help when
necessary may prevent unnecessary institutionalization.

Problems with Medications

One final class of problems for families caring for elderly
members with psychological disabilities at home focuses on
problems of drugs.
     Nurses and other health care workers assisting families
in their care of elderly members at home need to provide
information about medications which such patients may be
taking. Furthermore, nurses should assist families and the
elderly to develop safe storage, dispensing, and recording
systems for all medications.
     First, many older persons are medicated for a variety
of reasons. Diuretics, antidiabetics, antihypertensives,
nitroglycerin, and digitalis are prescriptive medications
frequently taken by older persons. Many older people are

also in the habit of taking a number of over-the-counter substances such as aspirin or Bufferin, laxatives, Bromo-Seltzer and Alka-Seltzer.

Many of the above drugs interact with each other, resulting in dangerous side effects. Furthermore, when these drugs are taken in combination with some of the medications most frequently used for psychological problems, even more dangerous side effects may result.

All drugs are potentially dangerous substances. The elderly react differently to more drugs than do younger persons. Furthermore, the effects older persons experience from a drug may change within a relatively short period. Therefore, it is of critical importance that the older person's drug use be carefully monitored by some health professional.

Drugs commonly utilized for psychological problems in the elderly include the drugs used for depression, drugs used to calm people, and drugs used for people who are psychotic or out of contact with reality.

Thorazine, Stelazine, Compazine, Mellaril, and Haldol are drugs frequently prescribed for persons who are psychotic. Some of the common side effects of these drugs (not as a result of interaction with other drugs) include: dry mouth, drowsiness, blurred vision, photensensitivity, constipation, weight gain, dizziness, headache, heat stroke, fever, sore throat, weakness, and decreased sexual interest. It is extremely important for a physician prescribing any of the above drugs to know if a patient is taking medication for hypertension, epilepsy, or thyroid disease, and if the patient has been diagnosed as having congestive heart failure, angina, or glaucoma.

Families should be aware that any of the above medications could cause confusion. However, before discontinuing a medication if drug-related confusion is suspected, the patient should be evaluated by a physician. Any person who is taking any medication, who becomes increasingly confused, should be evaluated by a nurse or physician.

Drugs frequently prescribed to calm elderly anxious patients include Librium, Valium, Serax, and sometimes Equanil or Miltown. These medications are taken by a large number of persons and unfortunately are not widely recognized as potentially very dangerous. Some of the side effects of these drugs include; dizziness, nausea, confusion, constipation, insomnia, stumbling, skin rashes, overexcitation, and decreased sexual interest.

Drugs for depression include Elavil, Tofranil, and Sinaquan. Some common adverse effects of these drugs are: dry mouth, blurred vision, urine retention, drowsiness, dizziness, constipation, headache, insomnia, and numbness and tingling.

While all of the above drugs have special interaction

with many other drugs, some general statements can be made
to assist families caring for elderly members who may be
taking any of these. First, combining alcohol with any of
the above drugs is very dangerous. Secondly, any patient
should report all known physical conditions and regular medications taken to the physician ordering one of the above
drugs. Use of any of the above drugs should strictly adhere
to recommended doses at recommended times. Double doses
should not be taken by a client if he happens to miss a dose.
Over-the-counter drugs, such as those mentioned in the beginning of this discussion, should not be taken without physician approval.

Finally, any changes in physical symptoms or behavior
of clients on any of the above medications should be promptly
reported to a nurse or a physician. If an older patient is
hospitalized, all medications should accompany the patient
to the hospital to be evaluated by the physician.

In summary, caring for older persons at home is a complex task. Nurses and other health-care workers must assume
responsibility for sharing their knowledge and their skills
with families and other caring persons who are motivated to
support the dignity and independence of their older members
and friends.

Below is a list of community organizations that may be
of assistance to families caring for an elderly person:

Visiting Nurses Association
Homemakers
Meals on Wheels
RSVP (Retired Senior Volunteer Program)
Foster Grandparents Program
Food Stamp Program
Senior Centers
Legal Aide
Department of Transportation, reduced fares
Public Health Nurses
Chamber of Commerce (list of businesses which give
        senior citizens discounts)
Churches, regularly assist members
Friendly Visitor Programs

References

Arling, Greg. "Resistance to Isolation among Elderly
    Widows." International Journal of Aging and Human
    Development 7(1):67-86, 1976.
Armstrong, Patricia W. "Comment: More Thoughts on Senility."
    The Gerontologist 18(3):315-316 (June) 1978.
Burnside, Irene M. Nursing and the Aged. New York:
    McGraw-Hill, 1976.

Busse, Ewald W., and Eric Pfeiffer. _Mental Illness in Later_
    Life. Washington, D.C.: American Psychiatric Associa-
    tion, 1973.
Cohen, Gene D. "Comment: Organic Brain Syndrome: Reality
    Orientation for Critics of Clinical Interventions."
    The Gerontologist 18(3):313-314 (June) 1978.
Epstein, Leon J. "Depression in the Elderly." _Journal of_
    Gerontology 31(3):278-282, 1976.
Grant, Elizabeth A., Martha Storandt, and Jack Botwinick.
    "Incentive and Practice in the Psychomotor Performance
    of the Elderly." _Journal of Gerontology_ 33:413-415,
    1978.
Green, Brent. "The Politics of Psychoactive Drug Use in Old
    Age." _The Gerontologist_ 18(6):525-530 (December) 1978.
Hellebrandt, Frances A. "Comment: The Senile Dement in
    Our Midst." _Journal of Gerontology_ 18(1):67-70, 1978.
Moses, Dorothy. "Assessing Behavior in the Elderly."
    Nursing Clinics of North America 7(2):225-234 (June),
    1972.
Patrick, Maxine L. "Care of the Confused Elderly Patient."
    American Journal of Nursing 67:2536-2539 (December) 1967.
Putnam, P. A. "Nurse Awareness and Psychosocial Function in
    the Aged." _The Gerontologist_ 13:163-166, 1973.
Schulz, Richard, and Gail Brenner. "Relocation of the Aged:
    A Review and Theoretical Analysis." _Journal of Geron-_
    tology 32(3):323-333, 1977.
Snyder, Loren Hiatt, Peter Rupprecht, Janine Pyrek, Sandra
    Brekhus, and Tom Moss. "Wandering" _The Gerontologist_.
    18:272-280, 1978.

CHAPTER 11

HOME-STYLE NURSING

Mary Kate House

Five years of training can qualify you for degrees in many
fields. By that standard, I am ready to graduate in the
area of unskilled and accidental at-home nursing. My prov-
ing ground is a private home situation involving an elderly
paralytic and two younger generations. Similar situations
must number in the hundreds of thousands (would you believe
a googol?) in the United States. I am writing in the hope
that my trial-and-error discoveries during these past years
may help even a few patients, "nurses," and their families.

Few occasions can top the day when your physician says
in a calm, matter-of-fact voice, "Well, there is really
nothing more we can do for him here. You may as well take
him home." You ask, "When?" totally unprepared for what
follows: "Oh, this afternoon if you'd like; we need his
room." Wow! You are picked up from the floor, while people look disgustedly at your "overreaction." But the doctor
says kindly, "Perhaps we could stretch it to a couple of
days." Well, Rome wasn't built in a day, but how about two?

Preparation

Now, about your two days--first think about a room. If you
are that rare family with a spare bedroom, skip the rest of
this paragraph. If your home accommodations are like mine,
start combining your living room, kitchen, and family room
into the handiest combination to free one room. Clear a
space for a hospital bed by a window that has the most
activity outside it. The bed may be rented, bought through
Medicare, or in some cases borrowed. You may do the same
for a wheelchair, if your patient can use one.

If you absolutely can't get a hospital bed, then put
concrete blocks or something sturdy under each bed leg to
raise your patient to a convenient height for bathing him,
feeding him, changing the bed, and all the other things that
have to be done for a bedridden patient. If you are using
a regular bed, you can order rails to fit it. Bed rails
are invaluable to your patient's safety; they are also a wonderful help in bathing him and changing the bed with him in
it. In my situation, the patient is able to cling to the
bed rail and lie on his side while I make up half of the
bed.

After the room, the bed, and the wheelchair are arranged for, your next move should be to get some outside
help. It took me ten months to figure this out, but I now
have the ideal arrangement. A neighbor (and lifelong

friend) is also a sitter at the local hospital. Our financial deal is based on the hospital's rates, but neither of
us sits much.

She comes in 5 1/2 hours a day, and we nurse, garden,
can, make soap, and freeze, pickle, and preserve food. We
swap our hours around to suit ourselves and to spend time
with our husbands, my 11- and 12-year-old sons, and my
recently married daughter and son-in-law. She does extra
hours on a given day to enable me to attend Little League
games, take one son to the orthodontist, visit our daughter
and son-in-law, and chauffeur the boys to piano lessons,
ball practice, school programs, camps, and numerous other
activities. I pay back these hours when she wants more free
time. Granted, our arrangement is exceptionally fortunate
for me, but there are other possibilities that I use or
know about.

For instance, our county has a nurse who will come in
free of charge once a week to bathe a patient and to change
a bed. Also, the immediate family can provide built-in
sitters. My husband and children are most willing, although
giving the patient a drink of water and a bite of candy is
about the extent of their nursing activities. Their company for an hour or so is a tremendous help. You should contact your local hospital, physician, county health department, Medicare, and units that specialize in treating certain
diseases. In our area some facilities furnish things like
underpads. As time goes on, you become aware of other home
nursing situations like your own and can trade help, advice,
and encouragement.

How to Change a Bed with a Person in It

This scared me out of my already scattered wits, but I promise you it is much easier than I can possibly make it
sound. Here is my trial-and-error method. It is quick and
easy, and it works. If your patient can still grip a bit,
roll him onto his side with his back toward you and ask him
to hold on to the rail. (Bedridden patients are delighted
to be able to do anything, even something this simple.)
Now push the used sheet and lamb's wool pad as close to his
back as possible, keeping the absorbent pad in place.

On the cleared side of the bed, on top of the air mattress, place a fresh double-bed contour sheet and fit the
corners neatly at the head and foot. Put the lamb's wool
pad on next, and shove it and the sheet close against the
ones that are being removed. Now adjust the rail on your
side to patient-gripping level. Roll him over to that side
and ask him to hold on to this rail. Go to the other side
of the bed, and slip off the soiled bedding. Pull the clean
sheet and the lamb's wool pad across the bed under him,
check the underpad for position, and then let him ease
back onto a nice, fresh bed.

     You learn a lot as you go along. It has taken me
almost five years to discover what a neat bottom sheet
the double-bed contour sheet makes, with a smooth cover-up
on the side most people see and plenty of slack to pull
through and smooth on the other side. If your patient can't
grip the rail, then roll him onto his side and draft any of
your children tall enough to reach up and balance him while
you get the clean bedding in place. If we keep the towels
and underpad changed as often as needed, we seldom change
the bed more than once a day.
     A list of bedding that has worked well for me consists
of three or more double-bed contours, three of more lamb's
wool pads, three or more twin-sized top sheets, and three
or more sheet blankets to use as top sheets when the patient
feels cold or the weather is chilly. If sheet blankets are
unavailable, buy four yards of outing flannel, cut it in
half, sew it together lengthwise, stitch the seam flat for
smoothness, and hem the ends   You should also have three
or more lightweight, easily washed coverlets, as many pillow-
cases as possible, and plenty of towels. These can be used
as bibs, sanitary pads, and for other uses. You can't have
too many, and the longer you use them, the softer and better
for your purpose they become. The extra covers can come
from the family supply. One of our cousins crocheted an
afghan for my father that is lightweight but snuggly, and
he enjoys it very much.

                         The Bed Bath

Now for the bed bath. Somehow, this didn't scare me, and
there isn't really much to it. You need a plastic or
aluminum washbasin, washcloths, lotions, rubbing alcohol,
bath powder, plenty of towels, fresh bedding, and a fresh
gown. Simply start at the top and work your way down.
Don't be too heavy-handed with the lotion, as it tends to
make the skin tender and more susceptible to bed sores.
Just use it on areas like the shins where the skin looks too
dry. You should bathe the patient just before changing
sheets so you don't have to be careful about splashing
water.

                       Toilet Facilities

These are, of course, an ever-present problem. My patient
is past being able to use bedpans and urinals, so I depend
on towels and underpads. To protect your mattress, cheap
shower curtains are the best thing. They look cheerful,
they launder well, they don't pick up odors, and they cost
about half the price of rubber sheets (which do not look
cheerful or launder well, and do pick up odors in addition
to their own smell, which isn't so great to begin with).
The towels can be changed quickly and easily as they get
wet.

Bowel movements are contained by the absorbent pad, which is always under the patient. We like the 23-inch by 36-inch pads best. They are thicker and can be cut in two. As they need changing, the patient can be rolled over to hold the bed rail until the pad is replaced. The dirty pad is pushed into a plastic bread sack; it is tied and placed in a small, tightly covered metal garbage can. As often as is needed, these are taken to a laundry hamper in the garage. This hamper is lined with a large plastic trash bag, which is lifted out and carried away with the rest of the garbage. There is no fuss, no mess, and little smell. The wet towels are put in a hamper in the patient's room and are usually washed in the morning when the bed is changed. Sometimes this must be done more often.

Bedsores Can Be Cured, but Prevention Is Easier

The laundry detergent you use is all-important. If a sore erupts, use cornstarch for applications between baths as well as for bath powder. Use an oatmeal paste in the bath-water. Shine a 25-W light on the affected area for 15 minutes twice a day. Antiseptic powder helps dry up runny spots, but we have found cornstarch more effective than anything else you might use. The greatest thing we have found for both prevention and cure of bedsores is an air mattress. A regular hospital type is best, but if one is not available, a plastic raft like those used in pools or camping will do. This rests on the regular mattress, under the sheet, lamb's wool pad, and underpad.

Diversions Vary with the Patient

My patient loves horses and broke his last one when he was 80 years old. From his long, venturesome life, he has many scars and souvenirs. One is a thumbnail that would do credit to a Texas longhorn. A hoof clipper is the only usable instrument for keeping his nail pruned back to a safe length, and he gets a kick out of this. In his opinion, any horse remedy surpasses a human one. (I do realize, however, that some patients might not react favorably to gall lotion, horse liniment, or hoof trimmers.)

Our patient loves any animals, and the children ride their horses up to his window. They bring in the dogs, cats, and rabbits to put on his bed--once, even a descented skunk. Another thing he likes is being surrounded by pictures of his friends, awards he has won, plaques that honor or amuse him. One of my father's favorite plaques reads: "All my visitors bring me pleasure, some by coming, some by going."

Television is also a marvelous diversion, as well as radio, tapes, and records. He loves reading or being read to. Our church brings home communion once a month, and Dad

enjoys this link with his church. People are kind about
visiting, especially if they feel their presence is a
pleasure.
      Eating is fun for some patients, and it is for mine.
He can (and does) digest anything. Treats of candy and
cookies help break up the long days.

Love Yourself

On days when all you do is clean up messes of various kinds,
you may feel like the last line of a mournful old spiritual:
"You'd be satisfied if you'd only wake up dead." Indulge
yourself. Never do the Christian martyr act. If at all
possible, find someone to come in for as many hours a day
as you can afford. Have family, friends, or a professional
give a once-a-week cleaning to your house. Believe anyone
who volunteers to give you a hand, and let them. Share your
burdens. Take care of you. If you have trouble falling
asleep, take a mild tablet that lets you wake up every two
or three hours to check on your patient but keeps you
relaxed enough to go right back to sleep after your check.
      Wear better clothes than you ever have. Keep your hair
done. Keep your weight down. This house-bound life and the
feeding of sweets to our patient is really rough on my
figure. Join a weight-loss club. My Weight-Watchers group
is fun and helped me take my surplus 20 pounds off (twice).
It presents a healthy program and advocates a philosophy
that applies to everyday living as well as weight control.
It gets me out once a week to meet new people.
      Go with your family to Sunday school and church. Enjoy
your time away from home, and don't spend a lot of it discussing your patient. Just make your medical reports
brief, thank the well-wishers for their interest, and go on
to greener fields.
      Choose your own diversions carefully. For example,
when you watch "The Today Show" and place names and general
excitement roll past you as you stay put, does it give you
vicarious pleasure, or does it make your relative confinement more irksome? You know your own reactions. Never
pointlessly put in time with television, reading, radio,
or any other pastime that doesn't make you happy. I prefer
gothic romances, mysteries, television comedies, and in all
cases, happy endings.
      Always milk the fringe benefits for all they are worth.
Nursing my father is invaluable as an alibi. It saves me
from committees, civic duties, serving as den mother, and
other worthwhile activities. My father is even a safe
bolt-hole from my own family. When the rest of my loved
ones are choosing sides for a good old donnybrook, I can
always pull a Florence Nightingale. I say, "Oh, Father's
coughing, I must run." I flap my wings, adjust my halo,
and go off to relative peace and quiet. I also feed my

patient during some of my favorite television shows and my
family, who would be interrupting the funniest part of
"Beverly Hillbillies" or the loveliest music on "The Lawrence Welk Show," waits until my patient is fed.

     See yourself as a person with class, individuality,
and personality. Do now wallow in grief or self-pity.
To quote Mrs. Emily Pollifax (one of my literary heroines),
"Don't try to bleed for your patient, just get on with the
job."

Note: Mrs. House's father died June 18, 1978.--Ed.

CHAPTER 12

HOME HEALTH CARE IN A RURAL AREA

Mary Elyn Lauth

Statistics show that rural persons are older, poorer, and
more handicapped than their urban or suburban counterparts.
Because most of the specialized and developed home care
services are situated in urban settings, the rural elderly
have an access-to-care problem.

Five percent of America's age 65 and over population
are homebound, while the percentage of homebound elderly
in rural New River Valley is 9%. In any one year 17% of
the elderly population can be expected to be hospitalized,
necessitating some additional periods of confinement to
their homes.

Statistics show that as their income level decreases,
the elderly evaluate their health status as decreasing proportionately. Although there is a correlation between self-
evaluation and medical evaluation of an individual's health,
self-rating tends to be more favorable. Those persons with
lower incomes tend to be in poorer health, suggesting that
they are less able to purchase the health care needed.
Therefore, the New River Valley Agency on Aging in southwest
Virginia, serving four rural counties and one small city,
implemented a Senior Homemaker Program in October 1977.
Funded by Title IX (Senior Community Services Project) of the
Older Americans Act, this service meets a dual need by providing employment for limited income persons age 55 and
over, who serve as homemakers, and by providing in-home
services to the disabled and ill elderly.

Title IV monies were used for a training program at a
local community college that included fifty hours of instructions in problems of aging, personal care, safety,
accident prevention, and meal planning and preparation.
Ongoing in-service training is provided monthly by our
agency.

A CETA grant provides funding for a registered nurse
supervisor. This R.N. is assisted by a social worker employed through a county CETA position who also helps in
case management.

Currently, fourteen homemakers are employed under the
Title IX program administered by the Virginia Office on
Aging, and four are employed through the Farmer's Union
Green Thumb, Inc. Homemakers work a maximum of 25 hours
per week, but the service is offered in the community eight
hours per day, Monday through Friday.

Homemaker duties are directed toward allowing the
elderly client to remain at home in safety and with dignity
and, when possible, to make institutionalization unnecessary.

Referrals are made to the Senior Homemaker Service by
hospitals, physicians, social and health agencies, friends,
and relatives. All potential clients, who must be over age
60, are visited, assessed as to need, and then a suitable
homemaker is assigned. Clients are charged a fee according
to ability to pay; often the service is free. Some clients
are served through Title XX funding provided by the local
departments of social services. If more extended homemaker
coverage is needed, the supervisor tries to help the family
find alternatives or refers them to the appropriate agency.
Our agency attempts to assist all persons contacting them
for service.

The Senior Homemaker Service has been well received in
the community, and a close working relationship has developed
between our Agency on Aging and the local social and health
agencies. This close relationship of health professionals
has helped in defining, detecting, and meeting other elderly
needs.

Our efforts to establish a homemaker service were primarily to prevent premature institutionalization of the
elderly. Other goals included reduction of expensive and
prolonged stays in acute care facilities, assurances that
elderly persons living alone would have a means of maintaining a safe and satisfactory standard of living, and the
provision of employment opportunities for the low-income
elderly to perform dignified and needed work.

When planning any type of home-based health service
for the elderly, questions of insurance and liability,
long-term versus short-term care, cost effectiveness, and
funding need to be evaluated.

Insurance and liability are becoming most difficult
problems. With our agency's homemaker service, we must
carry comprehensive automobile liability insurance, comprehensive general liability, workman's compensation, and,
possibly in the near future, malpractice insurance. The
annual bill for insurance is in excess of $2,000, signifi-
cantly adding to the hourly homemaker rate.

When dealing with chronically ill older persons, a home
health provider must come to terms with the issue of short-
term versus long-term care. Current funding for home services is based on the assumption that eventually a client
will improve and the service can be terminated. Unfortunately, this is an unrealistic expectation. Our agency's
Homemaker Program is serving 38 cases, 35 of which are
long-term. New home care agencies fill up very quickly
and long waiting lists become routine. There are no easy
solutions, although a minimum number of short-term slots
need to be maintained. Careful and continuous review of
cases will alleviate some of the difficulty but will not
eliminate the problem.

A third area of concern is cost effectiveness. Many
home health services show a higher hourly rate than that

computed for institutional care. The fallacy of this comparison lies in three areas: first, home services are
utilized a few hours or days a week; secondly, there is a
psychological comfort factor when a person can receive services in the security and protection of his/her home; and
finally, in comparing home services and institutional care,
we must think about appropriateness. Some persons need the
skilled and specilized services that only an institution can
provide. Others do not. What is appropriate and reasonable
for one case may not be for another.

Home services are expensive. In recent years, home
care services have been widely touted as a cost-saving measure. This may be true, although this issue is far from
being settled. Out agency's homemaker home health services
cost is about $6.90 per hour. Nevertheless, the utiliza-
tion of federally subsidized jobs and other federal grants
allows our agency to greatly reduce the actual out-of-
pocket expenses.

Despite our many difficulties, we know that home services, particularly those in the health area, are critically
needed. Statistics reveal that family and friends provide
over 50% of the service rendered to impaired older persons;
however, without the assistance of community-based home care
agencies, the numbers would continue to decrease. We must
capitalize on this natural support system. Today, rural
area local health departments are the major agencies providing home health care. These health departments cannot
carry the total burden.

The evolving Health System Agencies may help to alleviate this need by encouraging the development of home care
services. Area Agencies on Aging can then support the planning efforts of Health System Agencies through the funding
of home care service delivery agencies.

These agencies, together with the local Public Health
Departments and the Veterans Administration, can develop a
comprehensive network of home care services throughout this
nation similar to what is done in our area.

Our agency considers the homemaker program important,
because it does prevent premature institutionalization and,
at the same time, it frees expensive and overcrowded acute
care beds and nursing home beds. This program has allowed
84 disabled and ill elderly to remain in their own homes
with safety and dignity. In addition, it has provided
employment opportunities for 18 limited-income age 55 and
older persons who act as homemakers for our agency.

CHAPTER 13

THE MEDICAL DIRECTOR AND SERVICES

TO PERSONS IN AN EXTENDED CARE HOME

John O. Boyd, Jr.

With so many people interested in the administrative aspects of long-term care, perhaps we will find solutions to our many problems. In 1974 Health, Education and Welfare (HEW) began to require nursing homes to hire medical directors. At that time McVitty House had 301 beds. Today we have 327. Our policy has been to offer the best service to every resident at the lowest cost. This is a nonprofit home. Sixty-five to 70 percent of our patients are covered by either Medicaid or Medicare. We have been able to add to our services and have all that is required by HEW. We have a full-time physical therapist and a director of activities with the necessary credentials. Reality orientation has been a part of our program for three and one-half years. Maybe we can achieve the results that Dr. Folsom enjoys with people who have organic brain syndrome or senile dementia. We have a program in arts and crafts. We have a director of volunteers, but not as many volunteers as we could use. Our full-time speech therapist sees and evaluates patients with speech difficulties or hearing problems. Our social service department is composed of three women on whom we rely for solving the problems of patients and their families. Our full-time chaplain adds much to the comfort of our patients and their families.

Recently, the American Medical Association (AMA) printed guidelines for the medical director entitled Guidelines for Physicians Attending Patients in Long-term Care Facilities. It describes what is expected of you and will help those who have not had experience in taking care of these patients. A physician cannot serve a long-term care facility effectively without close liaison with a sympathetic administrator.

Not stressed in publications is the relationship of the medical director to the board of directors and the executive committee. Responsibility for the health care in the institution rests with the board of directors. The directors expect the administrator to see that standard is achieved. The medical director is responsible to the director or the administrator. We know the attending physician is the person who is going to be called first if a patient care problem arises. The medical director then steps in and assists the attending physician in any way he can. I will see the patient for him and report to him and see that his orders are carried out. Of course, sometimes an

emergency does not permit the contact of the attending
physician. Fortunately, our group of attending physicians allow me to go ahead and then, later, tell them
what has happened and what has been done. This is a
responsibility we have to accept.

The relationship of the medical director with the
nursing staff should be obvious. You must maintain rapport
with your director of nursing and her staff. Because aids
and orderlies render most of the intimate care of the patient under the direction of the charge nurse, close cooperation is essential. Your presence and your support must
be carried down to the aides and orderlies if you are to
be effective. One of the things the nurses wanted most,
when I came to McVitty House full-time, was to be relieved
of medical decisions. They had been forced to make such
decisions, because attending physicians were not always
available. Sometimes, patients were acutely ill and something had to be done. Now they call on me and they seem
happier and more secure in their positions.

Boards, and executive committees particularly, in a
nonprofit institution, have to balance their budgets. You
can't go in the hole. There is no one to bail you out.
They will discuss the "nuts and bolts" of the institution
and sometimes forget that care of patients is the reason
for the institution. Sometimes, I will stand up as the
meeting is about to adjourn and say, "Ladies and gentlemen,
our primary interest has not been addressed and you ought
to be appraised of so and so." They have patiently stayed.

One of our important ancillary services is a capable
dietary department. We have a dietary technician in residence and a registered dietitian who visits us several times
a month. We also have a food service manager. Every effort
is spent toward serving the resident the best food his doctor will let him have, depending on his diet. The other
day we had an order for a twenty-gram protein diet. A
twenty-gram protein diet is difficult to deliver. The only
way we can do it is by ordering bread from a bakery in
Seattle, which is the only place in the United States we
have found that bakes a bread that is so low in protein
that you can achieve a twenty-gram protein diet. We doubt
there is a hospital that could have provided the twenty-gram
protein diet that this doctor ordered and was very insistent
upon. Our dietary program is very important.

Rehabilitation to most people means the return of a
person to gainful employment. In the long-term care field,
rehabilitation is the regaining of any lost function, particularly, activities of daily living. When an elderly
person is able to feed himself again, this is a rehabilitative success. Through this multidisciplinary approach, we
have the opportunity to restore a maximum degree of function.

CHAPTER 14

MEDICARE AND MEDICAID: PROBLEMS OF THE EXTENDED CARE HOME

T. Stuart Payne

My sole experience in the health care field has been at
McVitty House. Success in managing has been due to prayer,
friends, and a dedicated board of directors interested in
health care. Managing McVitty House has been enjoyable and
is simple. Our qualified department heads accept responsibility and have authority to perform their duties. They do
their work and we watch everything run smoothly. However,
this is not the simplest thing to attain. The administrator's job is to coordinate and maintain the proper relationships, and to make sure there is no breakdown in communications.

McVitty House is a nonprofit organization. We do not
pay a fee to the board of directors. Only the employees
receive remuneration from McVitty House. We must take in
more money than we pay out. We do not have a sponsor as
do some nonprofit homes. We are not church oriented.

Other than spiraling costs, the number-one problem in
nursing homes is the amount of paperwork created by federal
and state governments when we participate in health care
programs. Until we are permitted to dispense with some of
the regulations that have no bearing on patient care, we
must do all things Medicaid and Medicare ask us to do.
When Dr. Boyd, our medical director, was employed on a full-
time basis, we received new regulations from the Department
of Health, Education and Welfare (HEW) which were interpreted
one way by our director and another way by our staff. We
found, when informing HEW of the ambiguous regulations, they
were then rewritten so that all understood.

McVitty House is certified for Medicare and Medicaid.
We have some veterans and some private patients. Some
things required by government programs are not wholly necessary. Necessity for Medicare and Medicaid has to be certified by physicians. Patient care should be certified, because we are spending taxpayer's money as well as billing
for private patients on Medicare. For Medicare, recertifi-
cation must be done within fourteen days after entering the
nursing home from a hospital. If you enter a nursing home
from your private home, you do not receive Medicare. You
must come from a hospital and must have been there at least
three days before coming to the nursing home. After fourteen
days the physician must recertify that this patient needs to
stay in the nursing home for extended care. Then he must
recertify every thirty days for Medicare and every sixty
days for Medicaid that this patient needs continued care in
the nursing home. Our monthly billings and medical

information sheets must be submitted to an intermediary, in
our case, Blue Cross. If the patient is certified as
skilled care, arrangements must be made to place this patient into a skilled care bed. Sometimes, this requires
several patient moves. We have 327 beds in McVitty House
and of these, 26 are certified as skilled care beds. In
order to receive payment for those skilled care beds, we
must have either a skilled care patient or a private pay
patient in them. If an intermediate care patient occupies
a skilled care bed, then we are not paid for it. In our
skilled care section, the patient care is the same as in
intermediate care. McVitty House makes no difference in
staffing of its skilled care or its intermediate care sec-
tions.

It is not fair to move an elderly person around from
bed to bed and from room to room. After an adjustment to
surroundings and nurses, it is traumatic to move a person.
There are sixteen states that have the "swing bed." We have
tried to get this in Virginia but with no success. The
"swing bed" would mean that in our skilled care beds, we
could either put skilled, intermediate, or private pay
patients. If they are "skilled care" and their condition
improves, in order to be paid, we have to move them unless
they are private pay patients.

If a patient comes from a private residence and is
admitted to the skilled care unit, no Medicare benefits are
paid. However, the patient or the responsible party must
be notified in writing by the facility that no Medicare
benefits will be paid. That's more paper work than we
think necessary. If patient is taken off "skilled care"
by the Utilization and Review Committee, the patient or the
responsible party must be nofitied in writing. Then the
facility can bill for three days, but only after written
notice. Sometimes, the attending physician might be out
of his office for several days. If we take one of his
patients off "skilled care," we send the physician a letter.
If he disagrees with the Utilization and Review Committee,
he has a chance to overrule their decision. Three days is
not enough time to give the nursing homes to bill for this
patient's stay.

Medicare requires daily nursing notes, whereas Medicaid
only requires weekly notes. Medicaid inspectors have told
us many times that daily notes are excess baggage. They
don't want to look at a patient's chart and see the patient slept well, the patient ate well, etc. They want to
know if there is any change in the patient's condition.

Medicare and Medicaid payments are based on allowable
costs for nursing homes. All nursing homes are entitled to
a reasonable profit. In order for nursing homes to receive
the proper pay for Medicare and Medicaid patients, they must
set a rate that is higher than what they project their costs

will be because Medicare and Medicaid will pay you either
your cost or your charges, whichever is the smaller amount.
At the end of the year, we don't want to pay either Medicare or Medicaid a large sum of money. Therefore, the fee
paid by the private patient is subsidizing the program
patient.

The doctor/administrator relationship must be harmoni-
ous if proper care is to be given. Often doctors are required
to do paperwork they think is unreasonable. We have to maintain good relationships with the doctors, because if they
don't do what the program says, we don't get paid. So far
we have been able to do this.

We are not opposed to Medicare and Medicaid. Today
65% of the patients in nursing homes in Virginia are under
the Medicaid program. Spiraling costs put many people on
Medicaid.

Nursing homes are trying to do a good job. For years
nursing homes had a terrible reputation. We know this reputation is improving. Medicare has required nursing homes to
be updated and the quality of care has improved. If they
are not doing their job, their license should be revoked.
There is a place in the health care field for the nursing
home owner who wishes to make an honest profit.

My friend, Walter Regirer, who is owner and administrator of a nursing home in Richmond, wrote the following
prayer:

> Heavenly Father, look down on us, your humble,
> obedient nursing home administrators, who are
> doomed to serve on this earth, taking care of
> the aged, the sick, and the convalescent, under
> the watchful eyes of H.E.W., the State Health
> Department, the Commission on Aging, a growing
> number of ombudsmen, and the public. Give us
> this day, divine guidance in guessing correctly
> when Medicare inspectors will make unannounced
> visits and on these occasions forgive us for re-
> moving from their sight a bedpan from the overbed
> table and picking up a meal tray from the floor.
> Give us wisdom to file our Medicare and Medicaid
> reports correctly on forms and under regulations
> which we do not understand. We beseech thee, oh
> Lord, to see that we may keep our jobs secure
> from an ambitious and aggressive director of
> nursing and, if perchance, we extend our rarely
> granted weekends off, have mercy on us, for our
> flesh is weak. Protect us from overdemanding
> family members who are browbeating our nurses
> and complaining to nursing assistants that they
> should pay less and receive more. Dear God,
> protect our employees from union solicitation

and lead them not into temptation for they know
not what they do. Keep them from asking for constant raises and forgive them not for their tres-
passes for they know exactly what they do. Make
our employees love us for what we are and not for
what we can contribute in salary increases. Grace
us with the solution to the problem of whether to
keep the doors in our nursing homes closed as the
security officers require, or keep them open as the
fire marshall requires. Oh mighty Father, keep
us ever supplied with oxygen and chucks, especially
on weekends and holidays and when our bed occupancy
reaches maximum capacity. Grant us the favor of
a certificate of need. This we ask in the name of
Joseph Califano, Dr. James Kenley, Blue Cross, the
Health Systems Agency, and the Joint Commission on
Accreditation. Amen.*

*With permission of Walter W. Regirer, Health of Virginia,
Richmond.

Part III

Communication/Hearing Problems of the Elderly

INTRODUCTION

Harold B. Haley

In an introductory paper Dr. Cantrell relates two brief
cases pinpointing the interaction of social, personal,
and anatomic aspects of hearing loss.

Mary Wolanin, a proficient, elderly communicator, outlines communications problems in society and their variations in different age groups. She explores the role of
the language differences and changes, and cultural components of communications. The communication problems
of physicians are recounted. From this general approach,
Mrs. Wolanin gives a second presentation on transmitting
and receiving messages and how transmission occurs by sight
and sound, touch and taste. She demonstrates the impact of
negative messages with their interpretations not recognized
by those transmitting such messages. Specific discussions
are given of communication with depressed persons and what
is needed for good listening.

Ralph Stoudt narrates the fundamental physiology and
pathology of communication. He outlines the functions of
language, speech and voice and discusses various hearing
aids and treatment.

Roger Ruth describes specific types of hearing problems
and their treatment.

CHAPTER 15

COMMUNICATION IN THE AGED

Robert W. Cantrell

This paper will introduce some problems of communication
in the aging. As a lad of five, I began to realize that
my grandmother, who had come across the prairies of Indiana
to Missouri in a covered wagon in the 1880s, had begun to
fail. Still very bright, she was having difficulty hearing.
She didn't get around quite as well as she once did. Mostly,
she sat sewing quilt tops. One day I was whistling as loud
as I could. She said, "Stop that whistling, it is going
through my head." I didn't understand why this bothered her
or that her hearing loss was due to aging (presbyacusis).
This "going through my head" is what we now call recruitment.
She went on, "Besides that, it is bad luck to whistle in the
house." I said, "Oh grandma, it is not bad luck to whistle
in the house." She looked over her glasses and without
missing a stitch reached over with her gold thimble, thumped
me on the head and said, "See there, it was bad luck, wasn't
it?" Presbyacusis, associated with recruitment, is a problem
in the aged. Hearing is an important part of communication.
However, nonverbal communication (the thumping with the
thimble) can also be a very effective form of communication.
    Years later a beautiful lady in her seventies, a former
opera singer, complained of being unable to sing as well as
she once did. As a practicing otolaryngologist I wasn't
surprised. Beverly Sills, an opera star, had just announced
her retirement and she still sings beautifully. Nevertheless, my seventy-year-old patient wanted me to solve her
singing problem. Examination revealed that she couldn't
tense her vocal cords. She was told her problem was due to
aging of the vocal cords. In an imperious manner, she
scornfully said, "Young man, are you insinuating that I am
getting older?" "Well, essentially that's what it is," she
was told. She asked what could be done and was told there
was no known operation or medicine that would improve this
situation. As gently as possible she was told the poor
analogy that you could run much better when you were
younger and you can't run quite as fast as you once did.
One month later she was back in my clinic with the identical
problem. Again, she was examined and her problem explained
to her. Again, she refused to accept this explanation and
left dissatisfied. Was it a communication problem on my
part? Then, it happened a third time. This time we sat
down and spent a great deal more time explaining her problem
to her. I'm not certain if she finally accepted the
situation.

People who are aging sometimes have a diminution in hearing. Some have problems with their voice accompanying the aging process. Finally, some have a general withdrawal when infirmed or stricken with some type of chronic disease process, and are not quite attuned to what is going on around them.

Organic or functional, aging process or disease, localized or general--these are the distinctions that must be made and treated.

CHAPTER 16

COMMUNICATION WITH THE AGED

Mary Opal Wolanin

As an overage-65 professional woman, my paper about communication with the aged in a health care setting is authoritatively written. The usual chronological landmark of age 65 is used when discussing our older people. Now, as part of that group, I offer my credentials as an elderly person. Aging is a relative matter, as any six-year-old who fears the big boys in the sixth grade can tell you. Aging is what happens to anyone who is five years older than ourselves. However, age 65 is so ingrained that it is the dividing line between later middle age and old age and instant senility. Our older people are not a homogenous group stamped out with the same cookie-cutter. No one fits a standard stereotype of the aged or the person known as Mr. Statix, the statistical mean of the aged from 60 to 100 with an average age of 75. Seventy-five-year-old people do not represent either the 60-year-old or the centenarian. Studies concerning aging deal with Mr. Statix, a statistical mean which ignores the extremes.

Now, the aging group represents at least two generations. When we are confronted with our own aging, that of our older parent changes our traditional roles of parent and child and even reverses them. We are two generations of older people tied by blood and kinship bonds that confuse us both. The younger member may take the role of the parent and the older parent may need the nurturing required by a child.

In our century, and everyone 78 years of age or younger was born in our century, which is also growing old, technological and political and social changes have occurred so rapidly that no five-year cohort will have experienced the same life history as any other five-year cohort. A man born in 1883 never talked over a telephone until he was in his teens. And he didn't see a motor car until he was 30, or a television program until he was 70. Man walked on the moon when he was in his 80s. But his son, born in 1913, never knew a world without cars, and he flew in the Army Air Corps in 1942. He has sat in front of the television set every Monday night during his 50s watching ABC. What we have not experienced tends to be history without reference points. For the man in his early forties today, World War II, World War I, the Civil War and the Revolution are all ancient history, but the 60-year-old had personal remembrance of Pearl Harbor, and his father of World War I.

Among the aged we have groups that have shared little of their total life experience and who have a generation gap between what Neugarten speaks of as the young-old and

the old-old (1). We can multiply this diversity by social
strata, sex, and education, and it is apparent the aged
represent the greatest range of human experience that it is
possible to know. In an earlier era, when change occurred
over centuries instead of decades, the elderly might have
shared a common life experience.

The pattern of family structure and relationships has
changed. Nineteenth-century man was not dependent upon his
children or on strangers for communication. He had a large
number of siblings and many cousins who had shared his life
history; communication was simple with his peer group who
shared his experience. Today, man is part of a vertical
family structure where he may be the survivor of all his
contemporaries. Families have become small. There is little
peer relationship with siblings or cousins, who may live
great distances apart. The older person may have no one to
talk with who shares his life history. Now, there is only
one person living who knew me as a ten-year-old, and there
are few who knew me before the age of 30. Those who shared
nearly half of my life are now dead. The common assumption
that all aged people can find a common ground is not true.
The aged, in the company of other aged, may have no true
peer group. There is a generation gap within the aging
population based on lack or failure of communication.

Communication problems have arisen because the rapid
changes have meant that each five-year cohort has known an
almost totally new world; family structure has changed so
that many old people have no one who knew them as children
or young adults, or even as young-old people. One loses
his life history when there is no one who shares it.

Today, among our elderly people we have the single
person who has no family. Such a person can only be seen
in the context of his family, but in this case that family
consists of the ghosts in his memory, and we know them only
when they are shared with us. They are there. The loners
write poetry in which they fantasize a loving family relationship they have never known. No man exists except against
the background of his family, even when that family is non-
existent. We have always been dependent upon the family to
be a support system. Much of our health care system is
based on the assumption that when the older family member
is in need of help, the family members are waiting with
open arms to nurture and cherish him. If the family is
the place where self-identity is constantly renewed, then
an absent family represents a crucial loss. Being a master
survivor has its penalties.

Our elderly not only have a different life history,
but their world has been so different from our own that they
have a different language and culture. Manners and customs
learned as children are pervasive and tend to be the stan-
dards by which all other manners and customs are measured.

The world we know through our childhood and our mother
remains the most important one. There was a reverence for
the elderly when there were so few of them, and when they
controlled ownership of land and resources that would be
inherited. Titles of respect were used. Older persons
address one another by the titles Mister and Missus rather
than by first names, unless they know each other well. But
any young person reared in today's first-name society calls
the elderly person by his first name. The older person
tolerates it and often has no choice; but he sees it as a
sign of crudeness and lack of manners and tends to distrust
the younger person. If he fails on the first yardstick, he
will probably not measure up on the other measuring sticks.
The four-letter words that are used so easily even on radio
and television were washed out of our mouths with soap by
our mothers. There are many word usages which we older
people have problems with. The young hippy character told
me, "For a woman your age, you are a very neat lady." I
knew she obviously didn't know the meaning of the word. She
left me wondering what an untidy person like herself was
trying to tell me. There are many words such as guy, gay,
and nouns used as verbs that confuse and frustrate those of
us who thought we knew our language.

In addition to the accents, dialects, and word usages,
we have another problem and that is the jargon of the
medical subculture. Most of us have not had a formal education. There is a wide range from Ph.D. to the illiterate,
but the majority of us never finished high school, and for
those who are age 75 and older, the 6th grade may be our
highest attainment. Many of us are self-educated. This
does not mean that we should be talked down to, or patronized
as is so easily done by those with great specialization in
some field of learning, but it does mean that the speaker
must use constant feedback to determine where his listener
is. For example: a phrase "decremental trajectory"
probably has no meaning for us. It is pure sociological
jargon. You would say "poor prognosis," but for those of
us who are doing it, just say "going downhill." We know
what that means.

There are no simple answers to communication with the
elderly. Each has had such a unique life experience that
each one is a totally different human being. But all of us
over age 65 shared this world in the 1910-1920 period.

We are trying to define aging in our society at a time
like no other in history. Finally, Dr. Rabinowitz of Israel
gives us a filter through which we can pinpoint the age of the elderly
person. He names the six ages of man: chronological,
biological, cognitive, emotional, social and functional.
He further scales each age according to the individual's
competence in handling stress: high competence, competence, marginal
competence and finally, incompetence. A profile of an

aging man on the grid helps to individualize a person according to his strengths and his losses. Few are totally incompetent in all six spheres and of the 24 possibilities there
are numerous permutations (2).

Chronological age means nothing as long as the individual is capable of functioning as a human being. The grid
allows recording of baseline data for comparison at a later
date. When an older person is profiled by competence, we
are forced to see him as a human being with strengths as
well as losses. This also gives a rationale for setting up
certain patterns of communication.

We have spent time defining aging in relation to the
process of communication. Communication is as abstract a
term as aging. We use the term so freely that we assume
everyone has the same meaning for the term. This is never
true for any idea. The old adage "seeing is believing" is
not true, and for the older person with his own system of
beliefs, it offers a big barrier. We have used this simple
three component model of communication to guide us in our
interaction with others.

                Transmitter------Message------Receiver
The naive assumption is the message is received unchanged
from the presentation in the mind of the transmitter. All
of us are well aware that nothing is simple, but operating
under the assumption it is has interfered with all communication, and certainly with the elderly who have much different beliefs, life history, culture, and even language uses
than the transmitter. My favorite communication model is
the Shannon-Weaver model that takes more factors into consideration (3).

Theories show communication to be composed of many
elements. Postman states that communication forms a system
by which people can establish a predictable continuity in
life.* It is dependent upon roles that are part of the
environment. Most elements in the environment are so
variant we do not see them until they are changed or missing.
The environment, including the people in it, is usually
consistent with our expectations. These roles we understand
and we depend on them to protect us in interactions. We
say, "He stepped out of his role," and we are expressing a
concern for an ill-defined situation. In the physician-
patient roles, we usually have a sense of invariance which
lets everyone get on with the business at hand. However,
when the individuals in that interaction are a young physician and an older person, we may have role conflict or
incongruence. The older person, who learned his relationships at the beginning of this century, has been taught to
see respect and authority lodged in the older person. The
young physician may have also learned that kind of relationship with his grandparents. The older person has a
stereotype of the respected physician that includes a

        * Neil Postman, 1976: Oral Communication.

Figure 16.1. Determining the true age of man by abilities to handle stress.

Levels of competence	Chronological	Biological	Cognitive	Emotional	Social	Functional
High competence						
Competent						
Marginal						
Incompetent						

Source: Drawn from concepts given in presentation by M. Rabinowitz: "The Six Ages of Man: Assessment and Clinical Implications." Paper given at the International Congress of Gerontology, Tokyo, Japan, August 22, 1978, by Mary Opal Wolanin and used with her permission.

Table 16.1. Shannon-Weaver model of communication

Information---Transmitter---(encoding)---Signal (message)---Channel (noise in channel)---Receiver (decoding)

Note: The adaptations to the Shannon-Weaver Model are based on Neil Postman's course in Ecology of Communication summer session course, 1976, New York University, CBS. The special problems of the aged were incorporated by M. O. Wolanin.

Table 16.2. Special consideration that communication with the elderly requires for the model

Information	Transmitter (signal)	Channel noise	The receiver
Generation gap in language and customs	Awareness of sensory deficits	Perception comes from within	Visual differences of the aged eye plus pathological changes
Level of abstraction	Is speaker's face seen?	Distraction in room noise or motion	Hearing losses of normal aging: loss of consonants and sibilants
Meaningful and relevant material	Do hearing aids aid?	Intensity of light	New words
Jargon	Do symbols denote role relationships? Change in role causes communication breakdown.	Ambiguity of signal or situation	Bombardment of sound
Older person's intelligence:			Hearing requires context
Fluid chrystallized		Expectations color what one hears and sees	Life History--culture and system of beliefs
		Needs control perception	Category fixation
		In abstract material the similarities are noted and the differences ignored.	Are categories understood and shared?
			Verbal behavior versus nonverbal
			Can new content be associated with old?
			Does anxiety, pain, fear, depression or loneliness interfere with reception?
			What is relationship that is expressed: equal, superior, inferior?

three-piece suit and a gold watch chain across his middle.
This just doesn't fit the bearded, long-haired young man in
casual clothing who presents himself as a physician and
calls the older person by his first name.

The younger physician works with the aged on the basis
of assumptions about aging. Not knowing, he must make
inferences. When we respond to others we use three modes:
as equals, as a superior, or as an inferior. In Samuel
Shem's House of God, we learn of interns referring to the
aged who just don't die as "GOMERS," an acronym for "Get
Out of My Emergency Room" (4). The tacit assumption was
that "GOMERS" never die. With this attitude, communication
with a "GOMER" can only be on a superior-inferior role with
the young intern assuming the role of superior.

Riggs has indicated that the University of Arizona
Medical Center and Southwest Arthritis Foundation has a grant
from the National Institutes of Health to help the young
medical student look at the arthritic in a new light.*
The arthritics are taught to be as knowledgeable about the
musculoskeletal system as the medical student. When the
student examines this patient, he is literally taught by
the patient. How does it work? The young physicians working under preceptorships are doing well in working with
patients and learning from them. The older physicians in
the community are having problems. Health care is a joint
enterprise with the patient carrying his fair share of the
load. Does this mean that he has to be treated as an equal
in order for therapy to be a joint enterprise? In addition,
there are classes under the same grant teaching the
arthritic how to talk with their physician. What is the
principal problem that brings patients to this class? It
is that they cannot get their physician's attention. At
our nursing clinic the patients complained more about their
inability to talk with the physician than of aches, pains,
and other symptoms. We spent hours with them helping them
to organize their approach. One woman said, "The only way
I can communicate with the urologist is with pus cells."
Another man told me, "I saw four doctors this year on my
annual check-up and not one of them sat down with me."
There is a failure in communication with the older person
struggling to remedy the problem. Are they expecting too
much of the physician in this interaction?

The older person is in an ambiguous and contradictory
situation. He knows he cannot respond as an equal and not
as a superior, so he becomes inferior. The use of metaphor
explains his answers to unasked questions. In order to
express his feeling of being inferior in the situation, he
turns to an authority relationship he has known during his
life history; he is the recalcitrant scholar before the
school master. He begins in an apologetic manner, "I hate

* Gail Riggs, 1978: Personal Communication.

to bother you--." If the physician finds nothing wrong with
him, he apologizes for intruding on the physician's time,
even for not having pathology worthy of note. Again, using
the metaphor of child to authority figure, if illness is
found, he wonders what he did wrong because illness is a
character fault. The metaphor is not one for which the
physician is prepared. If he accepts the patient's words
at face value, if he hears the content rather than the
relationship, he will be losing the real portent of the
communication. Metaphor expresses feeling and relationship.

In any message there are two submessages: content and
relationship. When content level is contradictory or not
meaningful, we tend to hear the relationship level. By his
whining, apologetic schoolboy manner, the patient is saying,
"What you are saying does not make sense to me; therefore I
am receiving only the authoritarian relationship between us
where you are the superior and I am inferior." No amount of
advice or "doctors orders" really penetrates at this point.
The physician's approach has been destructive of the patient's self so he resorts to the metaphor. Milgrim says
that when legitimate authority is present, relationship
overcomes content (5). Instead of the physician-patient
situation, place yourself for a minute in the role of the
speeding driver who has been pulled off the road by a traffic cop. His authority will eliminate much of content. For
a few minutes you will be the bad little boy who is dis-
obeying a father figure. Relationship is the only level
of communication in this case.

Also entering into any relationship are the categories
that we depend on to simplify the complexities of daily
life. We have to categorize to handle the bombardment of
data which come at us from all sides. The aged refuse to
stay in neat categories. Yet we try to put them into a
very few categories: the young-old, the old old, widows,
single, divorced, married, the disabled, etc. We try to
compress the last 30 years of life into a very few categories and use the similarities in these to guide us in our
thinking. The example of the "GOMERS" was one that demonstrated this hardening of categories or stereotyping.
Another is the assumption that all older people are candidates for senile dementia. The old couple were celebrating
their sixtieth wedding anniversary when they decided to
take a sentimental journey down to the old schoolhouse where
they had spent their childhood together. On the way home
an armored truck passed them, the back door flew open, and
a money bag fell almost in front of them. The wife picked
it up and hid it in an upstairs clothes closet. The next
day two FBI men knocked on their door and asked if they had
any knowledge of the lost money. The wife quickly said,
"No," but the husband said, "She is lying, she hid it upstairs." "Don't pay any attention to him, he is senile,"

the wife offered quickly. The FBI men turned to the husband
and said, "Suppose you tell us what you know about this.
Start at the beginning."   "Well," the old man started slowly,
"We were coming home from school and--."   One FBI man nodded
to the other and said, "Come on, let's get out of here."
     This story illustrates the pitfall of dealing with
the elderly. There is that label "senile" which has no good
meanings, only derogative ones. If the FBI men had listened
instead of using their hardened categories that include senility in the aged, they would have recovered the money. It
happened to me. I couldn't handle my luggage while traveling. Two people helped me, and their conversation with each
other showed me they put me in the "senile old lady" category. I needed help so I went along with it, but I wouldn't
want to live with it. I don't like to be treated as if I
am not only physically incompetent, but mentally incompetent
as well.
     We have discussed who the aged are, and found them to
be a unique group that cannot be approached with formula-
like communication. We have looked at communication as a
structure with context that may be more important than content when talking with the aged. There is one other aspect
which should receive equal time in communicating with the
aging person--that is, listening to what he has to tell us.
Listening is an important communication skill. The older
people complain that they cannot get their doctor's attention. Of course there is the threatening fact that once
an older person gets the floor he may not relinquish it
and the caregiver may not be able to get away. The unfortun-
ate truth behind all this is that what the older person has
to say, ask, and contribute is lost because caregivers have
rarely wanted to hear more than the answer to their questions. This is all right if the caregiver asks all the
right questions. There are ways of guiding the garrulous
into proper channels, but it must be remembered that the
answer he is giving may be to an important question which
you should have asked.
     To give a moment of absorbed attention while an older
person is talking is to give him a cup of cold water.

          T'is a little thing to give a cup of water;
          yet its draught of cool refreshment, drained
          by fevered lips, may give a shock of pleasure
          to the frame more exquisite than when nectarian
          juice renews the life of joy in happiest
          hours. (6)
                    Sir Tolfourd   1795-1854.

References

(1) Neugarten, Bernice. "Dynamics of Transition of Middle
     Life to Old Age." J. of Geriat. Psych. 4(1):71-100
     (Fall), 1970.
(2) Rabinowitz, A. "The Six Ages of Man, Assessment and
     Clinical Implications." Paper read at International
     Congress of Gerontology, Tokyo, Japan, August 22, 1978.
(3) Postman, Neil, Instructor. Course in Ecology of
     Communication, New York: CBS, New York University,
     Summer Semester, 1976.
(4) Shem, Samuel. House of God. Marek Publishers, 1978,
     as quoted in review by Edmund Fuller, Wall Street
     Journal, September 11, 1978.
(5) Milgram, Stanley. Obedience to Authority. New York:
     Harper & Row, 1974.
(6) Tolfourd, Sir Thomas Noon. Ion (Act 1, Scene 2). in
     The Shorter Bartlett's Familiar Quotations, edited by
     Christopher Morley. New York: Pocketbooks, Inc.,
     1964, p. 390.

Selected Additional References

Butler, R. "Man in Aging--Philosophical Basis of Gerontology
     from the Perspective of Clinical Medicine." Paper read
     at International Congress of Gerontology, Tokyo, Japan,
     August 21, 1978.
Cunningham, W. R., V. Clayton, and W. Overton. "Fluid and
     Crystallized Intelligence in Young Adulthood and Old
     Age." Journal of Gerontology 30:53-55, 1975.
Gribbin, K. "Cognitive Processes in Aging." In Nursing
     and the Aged, edited by I. Burnside. New York:
     McGraw-Hill, 1976, pp. 45-56.
Johnson, Wendell. People in Quandaries: Semantics of
     Personal Adjustment. New York: Harper & Bros., 1946.
Kalish, R. A. Late Adulthood: Perspectives on Human Develop-
     ment. Monterey, Calif.: Brooks/Cole Publishing Co.,
     1975.
Long, H. B., and C. Ulmer. Physiology of Aging: How It
     Affects Learning. Englewood Cliffs, N.J.: Prentice-
     Hall, 1972.
Riggs, Gail. Personal Communication. Member of project at
     Arizona Medical Center and Southwest Arthritis Founda-
     tion to Improve Medical Education and Patient Education.
     Tucson, Arizona, September 11, 1978.
Wolanin, M. O., and J. Pergrin. "Positive Health Education
     for the Elderly." Paper read at IXth International
     Conference on Health Education, Ottawa, Canada,
     August 31, 1976.

CHAPTER 17

WAYS OF TRANSMITTING AND RECEIVING

MESSAGES BY THE ELDERLY

Mary Opal Wolanin

Studies by Ayledotte showed that when personnel were relieved
of some of their duties to give more time to patient care,
the care was given to the more charming patients rather than
the people who were gravely in need of care (1). This shows
an important aspect of communication between health care
personnel and their clients, the patients. Communication is
a human interaction, and we tend to react as we have been
socialized to react, not as health care professionals. We
need patients who can hear us without our making a special
effort, who respond appropriately and who give us a warm
feeling of success while all of this is happening. We
usually think of helping the other person adapt to us. Can
the healthy young and intact health care professional look
at making adaptations which are also needed? We cannot pick
and choose our patients when we care for the elderly. We
meet patients whose problems in maintaining contact with the
environment are so great that they are frustrated and angry
and far from charming. We do prefer people who interact
with us on a pleasant level, but as professionals offering
service we cannot always make people change their customs,
manners, dialects, or speech and hearing problems to meet
our own needs. The real question is who must adapt? Must
the patients with limitations that may be insurmountable
adapt? Or can we also adapt? We have to stop and look at
our behavior in order to understand just what we are communicating in the communication interaction.
      When working with the deaf person as a group of novices
who interact on the 24-hour-a-day basis, how many times can
we repeat a message without getting querulous? Does the
message of annoyance on the face, and the turning away in
despair or disgust completely cancel out any sounds that do
get through the conduction system? Time is one of the
important nonverbal communications. We, who are so hurried,
often communicate by the amount of time we are willing to
spare to persist. Communication is the fourth most important survival need after air, fluid, and nutrition. We do
not operate on a professional level when we give up before
the patient does. In some fifty years of nursing, my
experience has been that the patient will continue trying
to get his message across if we can tolerate his efforts.
Who gives up first? The helping persons insist that
communication conform to their needs and not the patient's,
who read the handwriting on the wall or the impatience on
faces and knows when to quit.

Some methods of communication can take over when the usual verbal communication ends. We are all familiar with the wonderful art of mimes, who tell us their messages through pantomime. Pantomime is fun, and I have appreciated it most in foreign countries where my language left me in need of help. The patient who cannot depend upon words and word order to get meaning or give it must have felt the same frustration. Pantomime starts with the basic assumption there are certain things which we share: the need for air, water, nutrients, change of position, relief from pain, elimination, and human interaction of an affectional level, love. After all of these have been explored, then the real challenge begins. The next basic assumption is that the person needs to know what is happening to him and to have control over his own situation.

When communication by sight and sound are impossible and impairments are almost across the board, the time comes for interaction at the most basic level, touch. The tactile sense was the first to be developed by the fetus. It is the one that remains when most other senses are diminished or vanished. As a culture we have two positions. We either do not touch, or we have such rigid rules about touch that a little touch may be too much and we get in trouble. There are no-touch zones that must be observed carefully, but these are changing. The no-touch zones observed by people of my generation are disregarded by some of the younger generations and have disappeared entirely. A graduate student was experimenting with touch in nursing home patients. She tried hands, which are a neutral zone. The patients pulled away with tremors, so she decided to put her hand on the knee. This did not work--and for reasons that any woman over fifty could have explained in short order. The hands and the shoulders are zones which express warmth and affection and no threat. Outside of health care agencies, people shake hands when they meet. As health professionals we disregard this culturally affirmed greeting. The best physician I have known shook hands with his patients when they entered his office, or when he visited in the hospital. It gave me a feeling of equality that permeated our relationships in a very positive way. We don't shake hands with the wheelchair or bed patient. When seated by a patient a spontaneous action on my part is to reach and touch his hand; especially, when listening to him. No one has pulled away. One widow told me, "No one has put their arm around me since Ed died." Whether that was yesterday or ten years ago, it is too long. Here is a little free verse called "Minnie Remembers" whose writer is anonymous.

God, my hands are old
I was so proud of them once.
They were soft like the velvet smoothness of a firm
    ripe peach.

Now, the softness is like wornout sheets or withered leaves.
They lie here in my lap; naked reminders of the rest of
     this old body that has served me well.
How long has it been since someone touched me? Twenty
     years?
Twenty years I've been a widow. Respected. Smiled at.
But never touched.
Never held close to another body.
Never held so close that the loneliness was blotted out.
     I remember how my mother used to hold me, God,
When I was hurt in spirit or flesh, she would gather me
     close.
And my children hugged me a lot, but Oh, God, I am lonely.
Why didn't we raise the kids to be silly and affectionate
     as well as dignified and proper?
You see they do their duty, they come to my room and pay
     their respects. They chatter brightly. But they
     don't touch me.
They call me Mother or Grandmother, never Minnie.
My mother called me Minnie. And, my friends.
Hank called me Minnie, too.
But they are gone, and so is Minnie.
Only Grandma is here.
And God! She is lonely!

The important message here is not a hug but spontaneity,
which indicates human feeling and communicated relationship.
We have had that trained right out of us. Our teachers,
in their anxiety to help us with technical detail, forgot
we were working with human beings instead of pathological
lesions; that hearts beat with affection as well as blood.
Health professionals, who are unsure of themselves, do not
dare to let the patient glimpse a bit of feeling. I have
found it easier as I have grown older and experienced what
the older person asked. At a meeting in Apache Junction,
Arizona, an old man came up to me at the coffee break and
asked if he could kiss me. I practice what I preach. There,
in front of 300 people, he did what he probably had not
dared to do for years.

After touch, which is a quintessential human communication, eye contact serves to reach people. The frequent
interview position is at right angles to the patient. This
is not an eye contact position and for older people with
cervical arthritis, it may prevent seeing the interviewer's
face. Usually, the older person looks at the top of a head
bent over the record busily transcribing notes. Eye contact
can save the communication from being a failure, and it does
not take much. Two and a half minutes of eye contact during
listening has been shown to leave the patient with the
feeling that he is being heard and understood.

I cared for a very sharp elderly woman in the coronary
care unit. The great young cardiologist (GYC) walked in

with his entourage of a resident and an intern. She received
a nod of greeting from the GYC and then he positioned himself
in the right-angle position and the two members of his
teaching unit for the day stood on the other side across from
him. He asked, "Did you hear her S4 sound?" When neither
had heard it, he gave a lesson in finding the S4. The
conversation was between the teacher and the students; never
was the elderly woman involved. She turned her head from
side to side trying to learn what was happening in her chest.
The GYC turned and she frantically asked, "How am I?" "I
will have to look at your EKG," he told her as he left the
room. "What is an S4?" she asked, as she grabbed my hand
for support against the bad news. I explained what S4 meant,
and sat by her for a little while as her blood pressure
went down. A little later, a nurse came in and said she
could go home for the EKG was normal. She was almost in
too poor a condition to go, and the whole matter was a
communication problem.

One other sense is utilized in communication. This is
taste. One Christmas I took a hamper of fresh fruit to a
custodial care home in Tucson that was desperately poor,
a Mom and Pop operation. I watched the Pop of this home
take some grapes from the basket and slip the skin off and
then touch the lips of a blind and deaf elderly woman. She
grasped the idea and ate the cool slippery tart grape and
indicated she wanted more. I stood there and watched the
loving interaction take place between the owner and the
patient as grape after grape disappeared into that tooth-
less mouth. It was a picture of pure joy on both faces
and communication at a high level. Another deaf and blind
patient in the same building had "feelies" given to her.
"Feelies" are textured objects such as furry toys and smooth
and rough objects. The tactile sense versus the communication channel. The place was a dump, but not a dumping
ground, for it recognized human needs of which communication
is basic. Cold water instead of tepid, texture in goods,
and smooth clothing, which is freshly laundered and clean,
are important communication channels.

Also, there are negative messages for the patient who
cannot communicate with us in our own style and language.
Keeping a client waiting is one form of saying, "I dread
this interaction." It is always easiest to put the
unpleasant chores to the end of the list, hoping that somehow they will go away. The young interns, who named the
older person "GOMERS" (acronym for "Get out of my emergency
room"), are typical of this activity. The message comes
through very clearly to the person who waits and that
negative reaction quite overpowers any content of our
messages.

Mary Quayhagen asked open-ended questions of a large
sample of older people in an extended care unit (2). "What
causes you stress?" she asked. The major stress-producer

was personnel. Their comments fell into the following
categories:
    1. Cruelty--rough treatment--shoving, forcing tissues
into the mouth, sexual abuse of the patient.
    2. Crudity of language--discourteous language and
crude word forms.
    3. Dress--inappropriate and disrespectful. Dirty.
    4. Nicknames such as "Grandma" and "Gramps."
    5. People with little knowledge who acted authori-
tatively.
    6. Shouting and gossiping in halls.
    7. Lack of sensitivity of personnel.
    8. Negative attitudes of personnel.
    9. Lack of regard for patient's modesty.
The nonverbal communication implicit in these personnel
actions had been accepted because patients felt helpless
in the situation, but the messages had an impact which was
powerful. As care-givers we become so engrossed in treatment that we forget the person who is being treated. We
rebel against being mutilated, spindled, or folded. What
we do speaks so much louder than what we say, and can be
heard so well even by the deaf.
    Five hundred nurses were asked who they would rather
care for: the depressed patient or the comatose one (3).
Some 2% have indicated they would rather care for the
depressed patient. While 98% of us prefer to care for the
patient with whom communication may be nil. Why are we so
uncomfortable with the depressed patient? Remember, many
of the elderly's complaints are masking a severe depression.
They rarely admit it until questioned directly, but at some
point you are confronted with certainty. Depressed patients
never fall into the category of charming people. In fact,
we make the quick and, for us, comfortable assumption that
they prefer to be left alone. Communication with these
people is very challenging and words seldom carry our
message of help. There is no bluffing, but sincere touch
and presence tell of your concern. I had one patient who,
even in the depths of her despair, kept books on those who
had done something or spoken to her. She knew the phonies.
    Communication is a two-way process and listening to the
patient is the other half. How many of us are good lis-
teners? How many even want to listen? Are we afraid we
can't turn off the flood of verbage or feeling which will
come out if we start listening? Few young people really
want to listen to their elders complain of how they feel,
where it hurts, and, most painful of all, how neglected
they are. At the White House Conference for Aging in 1971,
the definition of "empathy" was "feeling my hurts in your
body." Can your body handle anyone else's hurts? Counselors whose lives are a tangled mess cannot help those who
come to them. First rule: be honest; if you are too tired
and impatient to listen, don't do it. It is only fair to

say to the other person, "I cannot listen to you now." And
tell them why. Older people are tough. They are master
survivors and they know all the things that hurt you and
understand. They respect you for honesty. But don't reject
by offering a fraction of a listening ear.

The second rule is abstinence. This means: don't tell
the older person to ignore what is bothering him, for he is
saying what he honestly feels. It may be threatening to you,
but it is a test of your own worth and strength to listen.
It is easy to give advice and ignore the feeling tone. The
older person knows that advice is the signal for the end of
the communication.

In conclusion, if you are uncomfortable in working with
the aged, in talking with people with impaired senses, or
understanding, or with the troubled people we are, take on
another kind of work. Life is too short to be frustrated
as those who have not mastered communication with the aged
are. There are other jobs which you can work at during the
time more skills and understanding of the many aspects of
this important form of communication are being developed.

References

(1) Ayledotte, M. K. and W. R. Hudson. "A Socio-Engineering
     Problem: The Nursing Profession." Nursing Outlook,
     10:(1)20-23, 1962.
(2) Quayhagen, Mary P. Confusion in the Elderly. Paper
     presented at the Chautauqua Continuing Education
     Seminar, Colorado Nurses Association, Vail, Colorado,
     August 3, 1977.
(3) Wolanin, Mary O. Unpublished study at University of
     Arizona, Tucson, 1973.

Selected Additional References

Archer, Dane, and Robin M. Akert. "Words and Everything
     Else: Verbal and Nonverbal Cues in Social Interpre-
     tation." Journal of Personality and Social Psychology
     35:443-449, 1977.
Blondis, Marion Nesbitt, and Barbara E. Jackson. Nonverbal
     Communication with Patients: Back to Human Touch.
     New York: John Wiley & Sons, 1977.
Bundza, Kenneth. "A Human Needs Checklist." Perspective on
     Aging 2:16-19, 1976.
Burnside, Irene M. "Touching Is Talking," American Journal
     of Nursing 73:2060-2063, 1973.
Frank, Lawrence. "Tactile Communication." Genetic Psychology
     Monographs 56:209-255, 1957.
Matson, Floyd W., and Ashley Montague, Eds. Introduction,
     The Human Dialogue. New York: Free Press, 1967.

Mercer, Lianne. "Touch, Comfort or Threat." Perspectives
    of Psychiatric Care 4(3):20-25, 1966.
Quayhagen, Mary P. "Adjustment of the Elderly to Institu-
    tional Relocation: A Conceptual Model." Diss.
    University of California, San Francisco, 1977.
Reusch, Jurgen, and Weldon Kees. Nonverbal Communication.
    Berkeley: Univ. of California Press, 1970.

CHAPTER 18

PROBLEMS OF VERBAL COMMUNICATION

Ralph Stoudt

America is getting older. The number of senior citizens is
increasing yearly. By the year 2000 some 29 million persons,
or 11% of the population, will be 65 years or older. We
are becoming more sensitive to the needs of our elderly.
This sensitivity is aided by formal and informal educational
efforts by the aged and others. Some would call this
lobbying. Attention is being paid to formulating responses
to needs of the elderly as need arises. Consequently, a
new way of life is being put together by and for older
citizens.
     Communication ability stands high on the list of skills
necessary for fullest enjoyment of life. The ability to
communicate is not only uniquely human, but also provides
means of conducting almost all our affairs of life. The
human community places a high value on communication ability. All of us feel excitement as a child passes through
the development of motor skills, from raising its head, to
walking without assistance. As important as those motor
skill milestones are in a child's growth, we are sure the
child has joined the human race when he begins to talk. In
subsequent years effort is devoted to making sure the child
develops his communication skills. At some point the child
becomes aware of the importance of communication in organizing and executing all aspects of his life. Language and
speech are then central to successful management of prac-
tically all of our affairs.
     When a person begins to experience some difficulties
in using communication skills, he begins to feel uneasy.
He senses his life can be disrupted to a significant degree
by communicative problems. As such concerns are experienced,
the person seeks aid in dealing with problems. The American
Speech and Hearing Association appointed a committee in 1966
to study the "Communication problems of the aging." This
committee had the responsibility of investigating those
aspects of gerontological behavior that contribute to the
disruption of communication in the aging.
     When communication is studied, it is necessary to
differentiate between language efforts and speech production.
Language is a system of symbols, a code. This code is
learned and permits communication between individuals. In
language, rules regarding grouping and sequential arrangements of those items that represent the code are learned
early in childhood. In acquiring a language code, there is
a genetic component present that makes the language learning
process possible and probably includes a drive to learn the
code. The genetic component permits most children to induce

from exposure to a finite set of language experiences in
their environment, sounds, forms, usages. This knowledge
of the rules of language make the child capable of both
understanding and creating an infinite variety of messages
in that code.

On the other hand, speech is made up of sounds and
sequences of sounds known as words. By making use of these
sounds, the child is able to encode messages he is generating
from his language capability. The terms "speech" and "language" are sometimes interchanged. When communication and
disorders of communication are studied, the differences
between speech and language must be carefully observed.

One of the greatest discoveries a child makes is things
have names. The production of the word, the coding of the
symbol that he has come to associate with the object, is a
speech act. The concept of the object, which he encodes,
is a language phenomenon. Children in other language communities set about coding their perception of a language
component in the speech they hear used in their environment.
The development of language and speech require attainment
of a certain minimal level of integrity of the central
nervous system and muscles of the face and upper body.

What does this excursion into development of communication in children have to do with communication to elderly?
Normal, efficient communication requires that the central
nervous system and certain parts of the neuromuscular system
be largely undamaged. Damage to these structures will
disrupt the communication function of those structures.
Communication disturbances may appear if the centers serving
language function in the left hemisphere of the brain are
damaged; such damage is considered to be a language disorder.

Communication disorders found in the aging can be
roughly divided into two categories, language disorders and
speech disturbance. The most common type of language impairment in the aging is brought about by arteriosclerosis. This
reduction of oxygen supply to the brain sets the stage for
appearance of a number of symptoms, among which may be the
disruption of language behavior. In his study of language
impairment in adults, Fred Darley of the Mayo Clinic labels
these kinds of language disturbances as language of confusion. Language of confusion is characterized by reduced
recognition and understanding of environment, faulty memory,
unclear thinking, and disorientation in time and space. All
of us have had the experience with this sort of language
disturbance. Insult to certain areas of the left hemisphere
of the brain results in another disturbance of language,
called aphasia. As cerebrovascular accidents are more common
in the aged, aphasia may be considered a partially age-
related disorder. Aphasia is an impairment of ability to
use and comprehend the conventional linguistic elements of
a previously acquired language system. One-fifth of adult

stroke patients have some persisting aphasic symptoms and
there are about one million aphasic adults in the United
States today, many over age 60.

In addition, speech problems may also be found in the
aged. Speech disturbance is faulty production of sounds
used for communication. The causes of speech disturbances
in the aged range from misarticulations caused by badly
fitting dentures to those caused by the loss of ability to
program sequences of movement necessary to produce communicative sounds. The loss of ability to program certain movements is called apraxia of speech. Darley defines apraxia
of speech as an articulatory disorder, the result of brain
damage in which capacity to program positioning of the speech
musculature and the sequencing of muscle movements for
volitional production of speech sound is disrupted. However,
one of the marks of speech production in apraxia is that
observed articulation problems are inconsistent. Further,
the same muscles that do not function properly in speech
production may appear relatively, or near, normal when
used for reflex or automatic acts.

Dysarthria, another weakness, slowness or incoordina-
tion of the speech musculature, is due to damage to some
central and/or peripheral nervous systems. In contrast to
inconsistency of articulation disorders encountered in
apraxia of speech, misarticulations in dysarthria are consistently present and muscle movements are impaired in
reflex and automatic usage also. Some degree of dysarthria
is familiar as a consequence of many brain disorders such
as Parkinsonism, multiple sclerosis, and others.

Another type of communication problem in the aging is
voice disturbances. A voice disorder is defined as any
deviation in pitch, intensity, or quality of voice that is
consistently present and consistently interferes in communication. Voice disorders are not found exclusively in the
aged. Voice disorders may result from abuse of vocal cords
such as hoarseness following an exciting football game.
Chronic abuse of the cords may result in the formation of
vocal nodules or other structural changes in the larynx with
more permanent vocal manifestations. For some types of
voice aberration, a period of vocal rest will contribute
to clearing the voice disorder.

There is another group of voice disorders arising from
organic changes in the larynx that frequently require
surgical treatment. Hoarseness is a warning sign of a
developing laryngeal cancer. The usual surgical treatment
of this voice-production problem produces the loss of the
larynx. Following removal of the larynx, the patient will
have to use some other method of producing sounds necessary
for production of speech. Some patients develop esophageal
speech, and others learn how to use some sort of sound
production device. Laryngectomy is not exclusively a
communication problem of aged, but it does concentrate in

elderly men. An estimated 9,000 laryngectomies will be done
this year in males whose average age is 62. This is just a
sketch of communication problems that may occur in the aged.

Some aids are available for the person or for the family
of the person with a communication problem. Many years ago
some "laryngectomees" joined forces and formed the International Association of Laryngectomees. The purpose of this
group is to provide a means of sharing experience and information that might help the patient and his family regain
confidence in his ability to communicate and to practice
new forms of communication. Modeled after the International
Association of Laryngectomees, there are "Stroke Clubs" in
some cities. The National Easter Seal Society has a pamphlet
that suggests ways a Stroke Club program might be organized.

In attempting to help nursing home staff better understand the communication problems of their patients, the
American Speech and Hearing Association has developed
materials to carry out an in-service training program. The
program is called "Breaking the Silence Barrier." This
association has developed a bibliography of materials that
may help families of persons with communication disturbances
understand the patient's speech and language problems.

CHAPTER 19

HEARING PROBLEMS OF THE AGED

Roger A. Ruth

Hearing loss is recognized as one of the major chronic medical problems. Approximately 20 million Americans, or one out of every twelve, suffer from some form of hearing loss. The most common cause of hearing impairment in the adult population is presbyacusis, defined as hearing loss related to advancing age. Presbyacusis is also one of the least understood forms of hearing impairment. Diagnosis is usually made on the basis of ruling out other identifiable causes in the presence of old age. Presbyacusis is not now medically treatable, but if identified, steps can be taken to reduce the overall impairment through the use of hearing aids and other rehabilitative procedures.

Presbyacusis in varying degrees affects approximately 60% of the nearly 20 million individuals now over age 65. Furthermore, the overall number of individuals with presby-acusis is expected to increase based on current estimates of increases in life expectancy.

Inability to communicate effectively with one's environ-ment as a result of hearing loss can have a devastating impact leading to social withdrawal and increased emotional stress. The health care professionals who deal with elderly persons should be aware of the complications that can arise from this form of hearing impairment.

Presbyacusis is manifested as a slow progressive deter-ioration of hearing that becomes noticeable beyond age 65. The physiological processes responsible for this deteriora-tion in hearing ability are likely present almost from birth. The frequency range to which the human ear will respond re-mains fairly constant from about 20 to 20,000 Hz (Hertz, or cycles per second) through the second decade of life. Beyond age 20 there begins a gradual decrease in hearing sensitivity from the upper portion of this range toward lower frequencies. For example, a 30-year-old individual might be expected to have an upper frequency limit of around 15,000 Hz instead of 20,000 Hz, and a forty year old person may be able to hear only sound with frequencies below 12,000 Hz.

Routine clinical hearing measurement makes use of tones selected in octave steps between 250 Hz and 8,000 Hz. This group of frequencies represents a region of sound energy most critical to speech perception, which is the primary function of the human ear. Most of the sound energy con-tained in the speech signal is between 300 Hz and 3,000 Hz. Because of this, the gradual loss of high frequency hearing (above 8,000 Hz) goes virtually unnoticed to all but the most experienced audiophile.

Figure 19.1

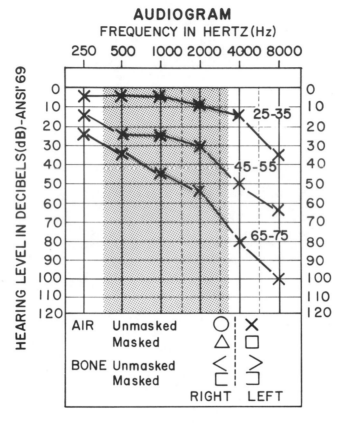

Audiogram illustrating relative hearing ability for
tones as a function of age.

The audiometric curves shown in Figure 19.1 exhibit
the tendency for increasing loss of hearing with advancing
age.   These curves represent a theoretical average hearing
sensitivity for men.   There is a definite sex difference
seen in individuals with presbyacusis, with females being
less affected than males.   The most frequent explanation
offered for these differences is that males are more likely
than females to have been exposed to hazardous occupational
and recreational noise.   Noise exposure produces a high
frequency hearing loss and, therefore, may combine with the
aging process to augment the total hearing loss.
     Certain medications, such as salicylates, aminoglycos-
ides, diuretics, and some anticancer agents, are known to
produce changes in the auditory mechanism.   Since many of

these agents are used in the treatment of various diseases
which affect the elderly, any hearing loss observed may be
a result in part of ototoxicity.

Presbyacusis typically affects both ears to a similar
extent. There is an element of individual susceptibility
involved in that some 80-year-old individuals have little
evidence of hearing loss, whereas persons as young as 50
years may exhibit a significant hearing impairment. There
may also be a genetic predisposition for this form of hearing loss, since presbyacusis is more prevalent in some
families than others.

The pathophysiology associated with presbyacusis is
extremely complex and not now well understood. Apparently,
impairment results from structural changes that occur
throughout the entire auditory system including the outer,
middle, and inner ear and central nervous pathways. Hearing
loss from presbyacusis is predominately of the sensorineural
type. Therefore, the contribution of the outer and middle
ear is considered minimal. Presbyacusis, no doubt, results
from an accumulation of degenerative processes of the sensory organ and its central pathways.

A primary concern associated with any form of hearing
impairment is the degree to which speech perception will be
affected. As indicated earlier, presbyacusis generally
manifests a high frequency hearing loss with relatively
normal hearing for low frequencies. The consonant sounds
contributing to the intelligibility of the speech signal
contain high frequency energy (1,000 Hz to 4,000 Hz). Thus,
a reduction of hearing sensitivity at these same frequencies
can cause a relative reduction in speech discrimination.
The following example will illustrate the effect of removal
of certain consonant sounds in an utterance as well as a
result of high frequency hearing loss:

Normal: Our office is on the twelfth floor.
High frequency hearing loss: Our o_ i e i_ on __e
we l___ loor.

That is why many individuals with presbyacusis express the
following complaint: "I can hear you, but I can't understand you."

Some individuals experience a drastic reduction in
speech-discrimination ability disproportionate to the degree
of pure tone sensitivity loss. This impairment, known as
phonemic regression, occurs less frequently and is believed
to be a result of degeneration in the central auditory pathways. As such, it poses a more serious problem to successful
rehabilitation.

It was long believed that individuals with presbyacusis
could not benefit from the use of a hearing aid. This was
because early forms of hearing aids were unable to selec-
tively amplify the high frequencies without also amplifying
the lows. With improved hearing aid design, it is possible
to tailor the hearing aid characteristics to the needs of

the patient. As a result, the majority of persons with
presbyacusis can now benefit from using hearing aids.
However, because of the complexity of this hearing impairment, providing satisfactory amplification to the patient
represents a significant challenge. It is not sufficient
to recommend the purchase of a hearing aid based on the
identification of a hearing loss without regard for the
specific auditory capabilities and motivation of the client.
Purchase of a hearing aid is justified only if it is worn
and properly used. Dissatisfaction with the hearing aid
often results from a lack of understanding of its limitations and from a lack of knowledge of its use.

A more extensive evaluation beyond the basic hearing
test is required to determine the most suitable form of
amplification for the patient. Measures obtained during
this examination permit the specification of various parameters of the hearing aid such as frequency response,
degree of amplification, and maximum output. Some individuals with presbyacusis experience a loudness-tolerance
problem resulting in an inability to withstand sounds
amplified beyond a certain level. In order to accommodate
this problem, the hearing aid may be adjusted by various
methods in order to limit its maximum output. The presence
of a severe tolerance problem may in fact preclude the use
of a hearing aid altogether.

A second phase of the evaluation procedure designed to
further assess the success of the hearing aid fitting,
relies on an extended trial period (usually one to two months
months). The patient wears the aid in a variety of everyday
situations germane to his or her environment. During the
trial period the patient returns to the clinic for additional assessment and counseling. This visit reorients the
individual as to the proper use of the hearing aid as well
as provides an opportunity to make any adjustments necessary
for optimal utilization.

Aural rehabilitation therapy will be of benefit to many
individuals with presbyacusis. Lip-reading skills allow
maximal utilization of visual cues that may enhance speech
discrimination ability. Family members are often included
in this therapy program to promote their understanding of
the specific impairment and its consequences, and facilitate the client's carry-over of acquired lip-reading skills
into the home environment.

Hearing impairment observed in presbyacusis need not
be the cause of social isolation for the elderly person.
Early identification of the hearing loss and skillful
management of the rehabilitation program will allow the
individual to compensate effectively. The participation
of family members in the program cannot be overemphasized,
as their support is often necessary for its success.

Part IV

Nutrition and the Elderly

INTRODUCTION

Harold B. Haley

What are the nutritional needs of the elderly? Are they different from the needs of the younger or the middle-aged person? Sanford Ritchey relates causes of poor food habits. He describes the decrements in physiological parameters that occur in aging. Specific problems of obesity are discussed. Requirements for protein, vitamins, minerals, and iron are listed.

Marilyn Donato explains how to take a diet history and presents an outline used in taking such histories. She presents various nutritional abnormalities with their causes and practical solutions. Costs of obtaining good nutrition are analyzed and practical tips given to hold down costs.

Janet Austin shows how nutritional care should be applied to individual patients in the hospital setting and emphasizes the personal role of the care-giver.

Sidney Barritt, a gastroenterologist, presents the gut functions in an elderly person. He describes the various medical situations which affect nutrition, including gastrointestinal tract surgery, cutting of the vagus nerve, hernias, by-pass operations for obesity, the use of antacids, alcohol, various medications (digitalis causing anorexia being an important one), and then other illness conditions, such as congestive heart failure and dyspnea. All of these impinge on the nutritional state. In many cases, we have very little knowledge of long-standing effects of medications, illnesses, or operations and what these can do to the nutritional state.

CHAPTER 20

NUTRITION OF THE ELDERLY

Sanford J. Ritchey

Many nutritional problems of the elderly result from a history of poor food habits. Good nutrition practices can prevent occurrences of certain physiological problems and delay the onset of others. Poor habits of food consumption can lead to the early onset of cardiovascular maladies, diabetes, hypertension, obesity, osteoporosis, and dental caries.

As a person ages, loss of teeth and/or poor-fitting dentures and decreasing sensitivity of taste and smell interfere with utilization of food and may influence food intake. These alter dietary habits of the elderly. Many elderly persons will adopt a soft diet, high in carbohydrates and low in protein and other nutrients. Food may become less appealing and monotonous, and an adequate diet is not consumed.

Physiological performance declines with aging and may be influenced by and affect nutritional needs of the elderly (1). The following decrements (Figure 20.1) are well established. Decreases of function between age 30 and 80, expressed on a percentage basis are: (1) fasting blood glucose--no decline, (2) nerve conduction and activity of cellular enzymes -17%, (3) resting cardiac index -30%, (4) vital capacity and renal blood flow -50%, (5) maximum breathing capacity -60%, and (6) maximum work rate and oxygen uptake -70%.

The loss of muscle mass during aging represents an example of the decline in number of cells (2). Body potassium concentration, an index of cells, decreases significantly in both males and females (Figure 20.2)

Both body weight and thickness of skinfold also decline with age, reflecting a loss of muscle mass and decreases in body fat (Figure 20.3).

The decline in body size and cellular mass is reflected in nutritional need for energy. The total energy need of an individual is the result of energy expenditures for basal metabolism and activity (3). Basal metabolism declines significantly with age (Figure 20.4).

Basal metabolism has been defined as energy required to maintain essential process of life. The energy required to maintain life thus decreases from approximately 42 kcals at age 15 to 33 kcals at age 80 per unit of body mass (in this example, per square meter of body surface).

In addition to the decline in maintenance requirements for energy, the activity level declines with age.

These widely quoted data show that the energy expenditure reported by men decreases from 1175 kcals/day to 640

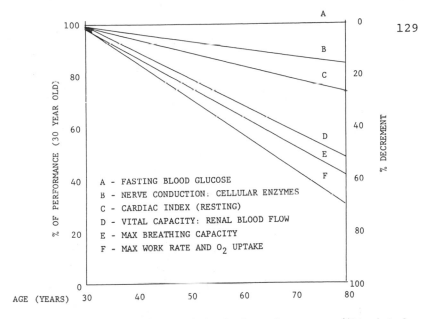

A - FASTING BLOOD GLUCOSE
B - NERVE CONDUCTION: CELLULAR ENZYMES
C - CARDIAC INDEX (RESTING)
D - VITAL CAPACITY: RENAL BLOOD FLOW
E - MAX BREATHING CAPACITY
F - MAX WORK RATE AND O_2 UPTAKE

Figure 20.1. Age decrements in physiological performance. (Reprinted from Developmental Physiology and Aging, Copyright © 1972, P. S. Timiras, with permission of the publisher, The Macmillan Company, New York.)

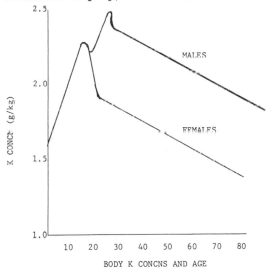

Figure 20.2. Potassium concentration of the human body as a function of age. (Reprinted from Anderson, E. C., and W. H. Langham, Science 130:713-714, 18 September, 1959 with permission of the publisher, American Association for the Advancement of Science.)

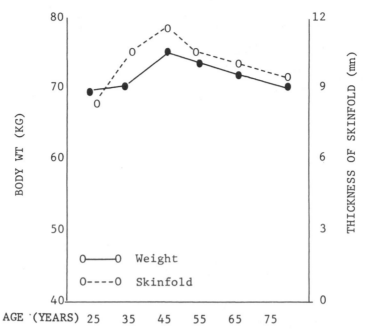

Figure 20.3. Changes with age in body weight and subcutaneous fat.
(Reprinted from Developmental Physiology and Aging,
Copyright © 1972, P. S. Timiras, with permission of the
publisher, The Macmillan Company, New York.)

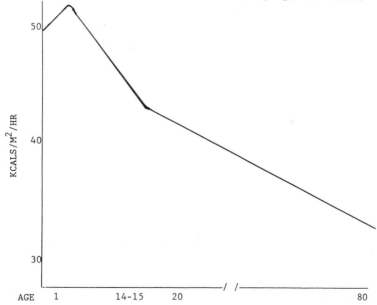

Figure 20.4. Basal metabolism as a function of age.

kcals/day as they age from young adults (20-34 years of age)
to elderly (above 74 years of age). Thus, it appears that
total energy needs decline with age (4).

Caloric intake and inactivity are related to obesity,
a major problem in our population. Obesity is the accumulation of excess fat in body tissues and is usually the result
of excess consumption of calories. In most adults obesity
results from long-term excesses, rather than the gaining of
weight over a short time span. Many people may gain from
three to five pounds per year, but when this occurs over a
20- to 25-year period there is significant weight gain.
Many elderly persons may be obese because of food habits of
a lifetime. Should an elderly person begin a program of
weight reduction, careful dietary counseling will be necessary. An elderly person will not be physically able to
increase the level of exercise to expend large amounts of
energy; thus intake of calories appears to be proper control. Elderly persons should not attempt to accomplish
weight loss prior to consultation with a physician and under
supervision of a dietitian.

Utilization of protein from foods is not a problem from
a physiological viewpoint. The nutrition literature men-
tions that the elderly may utilize protein less efficiently,
and their dietary requirements may be different from young
adults. The 1974 Recommended Daily Allowances (5) for
protein by the adult over 50 years of age is 56 grams for
males and 46 grams for females. For both sexes this
recommended intake is only slightly different from that
of the young adult. The protein allowance is based upon a
figure of 0.47 grams of protein per kilogram of body weight
per day. Usually, protein needs can be met if protein
represents from 10%-15% of total calorie intake. Most
nutrition scientists agree that additional research is
needed to understand the protein and amino acid needs of
individuals throughout life (6).

The 1974 Recommended Daily Allowances of Nutrients
with emphasis on the older adult population is shown in
Table 20.1. These recommended allowances remain constant
throughout adult life. Thus, physiological needs do not
change during adult years, except for periods of quite
different functions, such as pregnancy and lactation (7).
These allowances may reflect our ignorance about changing
nutritional needs with aging. However, based on present
knowledge and judgments of nutrition scientists, the vitamin
needs remain unchanged. The National Nutrition Survey (8)
indicated that many elderly persons were deficient in
vitamins A and C.

Table 20.1. Recommended daily allowances for adults above 50 years
            of age

Nutrient	Male	Female
Energy (kcals)	2400.0	1800.0
Protein (g)	56.0	46.0
Vitamin A (IU)	5000.0	4000.0
Vitamin D (IU)	400.0	400.0
Vitamin C (mg)	45.0	45.0
Riboflavin (mg)	1.5	1.1
Thiamin (mg)	1.2	1.0
Calcium (mg)	800.0	800.0
Iron (mg)	10.0	10.0
Zinc (mg)	15.0	15.0

Source: Recommended Dietary Allowances, Food and Nutrition Board,
         National Academy of Sciences, Washington, D.C., 1974.

     Though the elderly may be prone to low intakes of
vitamins, vitamin supplementation might not be required
for all. Supplementation may only be beneficial to certain
individuals. One survey has demonstrated that elderly persons were consuming supplements that failed to provide the
missing diet nutrients (9). Dietary counseling can be helpful in avoiding those mistakes and can result in money
savings for the individual.
     Most minerals seem to present fewer problems. This
may reflect our ignorance of nutritional requirements and
good evaluative parameters. Two minerals are worth a brief
discussion. Calcium is often cited as being low in adult
diets, and there is a high incidence of osteoporosis, or
decalcification of bone, in the older adult. This physical
problem may reflect long-term low intakes of calcium and/or
the particular combination of nutrients throughout life (10).
Females are prone to osteoporosis. From a physiological
view, the decalcification seems to be a part of the normal
aging process and will occur regardless of nutrition. However, proper nutrition throughout life and during the period
of bone development may be significant in delaying and
retarding decalcification.
     Iron-deficiency anemia is recognized as a prevalent
nutritional problem. The deficiency is prominent in females
during childbearing years or during the time there is
regular loss of blood during the menstrual cycle. The

recommended allowance for iron drops from 18 to 10 mg daily
as women reach menopause. There is poor utilization of iron.
Supplementation may be appropriate in some cases, but counseling is recommended before this is initiated.

In summary, important points need to be made in relation
to the nutritional health of the elderly:

1. The elderly tend to pay the price or reap rewards
for long-term food habits.

2. Nutritional problems may be different for the
elderly because of associated decreased biological function.

3. The elderly can benefit from good dietary counseling and should utilize those services before changing diet
patterns, using supplements or purchasing "fad" foods.

4. Nutritional requirements of the elderly are not
well known. Consequences of dietary patterns on the aging
process and on the complications of the elderly are not well
understood.

5. The nutritional needs of the elderly, as well as
other population groups, are related to a host of social and
economic factors.

References

(1) Timiras, P. S. Developmental Physiology and Aging.
     New York: Macmillan, 1972.

(2) Anderson, E. C., and W. H. Langham. "Average Potas-
     sium Concentration of the Human Body as a Function of
     Age." Science 130:713, 1959.

(3) Shock, N. W. "Energy Metabolism, Caloric Intake and
     Physical Activity of the Aging." In Nutrition in Old
     Age, edited by L. A. Carlson. Uppsala, Sweden:
     Almquist and Wiksell, 1972, pp. 12-23.

(4) McGandy, R. B., C. H. Barrows, J. A. Spanias, A.
     Meredith, J. L. Stone, and A. R. Morris. "Nutrient
     Intakes and Energy Expenditures in Men of Different
     Ages." J. Gerontology 21:581-587, 1966.

(5) Food and Nutrition Board. Recommended Dietary
     Allowances. 8th ed. Washington, D.C.: National
     Academy of Sciences, 1974.

(6) Munro, H. H. "Protein Requirements and Metabolism
     in Aging." In Nutrition in Old Age, edited by L. A.
     Carlson. Uppsala, Sweden: Almquist and Wiksell, 1972,
     pp. 32-45.

(7) Darke, S. J. "Requirements for Vitamins in Old Age."
     In Nutrition in Old Age, edited by L. A. Carlson.
     Uppsala. Sweden: Almquist and Wiksell, 1972, pp.
     107-117.

(8) Center for Disease Control. Ten-State Nutrition Survey,
     1968-1970. DHEW Publ. no. (HSM) 72-8134, Washington,
     D.C.: Health Services and Mental Health Administration,
     1972.

(9)   Todhunter, E. N.   "Life Style and Nutrient Intake in
       the Elderly."   In Nutrition and Aging, edited by M.
       Winick.   New York: John Wiley & Sons, 1976, pp. 118-127
(10)   Lutwak, L.   "Periodontal Disease."   In Nutrition and
       Aging, edited by M. Winick.   New York: John Wiley &
       Sons, 1976, pp. 145-153.

CHAPTER 21

NUTRITIONAL CARE FOR THE ELDERLY

Marilyn Donato

Nutritional care for the elderly can be practical and easily obtained. The older the person, the longer and more complex his dietary history. Nutritional status is the result of heredity, environment, and food habits throughout life. Therefore, the nutritional requirements of the elderly need to be more individualized when a therapeutic diet is indicated. Their food habits do not always coincide with their food needs. Many of us know how difficult it is to alter food habits. However, this is not impossible. When trying to improve an older person's food habits, "Never too old to learn" is a far truer adage than "You can't teach an old dog new tricks."

Taking a diet history is one of the elementary tools in assessing their nutritional state. Establishing rapport with the person supplying the diet history information is essential to gathering accurate information.

Table 21.1 shows a form suitable for taking a diet history that can double as a food intake record. The four basic food groups: milk, meat, fruit and vegetables, and bread are listed. There is space for recording diet intake for three days. For instance, if on Day 1 the person drank 2 cups of milk, two check marks would be placed beside the milk group in the Day 1 column. This process would be repeated for each of the food groups on each of the diet survey days. An average diet intake is calculated for each food group and compared to the recommended minimums. If the average falls below the recommended minimums, you would be able to determine whether or not the person's nutritional habits were meeting the dietary requirements. This form is useful in the practice of clinical dietetics.

Nutritional surveys of the elderly have shown the following problems.

1. Calcium deficiency is a common finding. This deficiency is probably due to insufficient consumption of calcium-enriched foods or the presence of endocrine abnormality. There may be poor calcium absorption because of lowered gastric acidity, or there might be hepatic and pancreatic insufficiency. Lack of exposure to sunlight, causing low Vitamin D storage, could also result in calcium deficiency. Practical solutions may include increasing calcium intake from 0.8 grams to 1 gram daily. Two cups of milk or yogurt give approximately 600 mg. of calcium, and a cup of salmon with bones yields approximately 500 mg. of calcium. Another practical solution might be calcium supplementation if all other natural sources cannot be used.

Table 21.1. Taking a diet history.

DIET HISTORY

Name:

Age:_____ Wt:_____ Ht:_____ Date:_____

Address:

Food Group	Portion size considered one serving	Day 1	Day 2	Day 3	Average	Recommended Minimums	Differe
						60+ yr	
MILK	1 C. (8 oz.) milk, yogurt. 1½ oz. cheddar, proces. cheese 1½ C. cottage cheese					2	
MEAT	2-3 oz. cooked lean meat, fish, poultry 2 eggs 4 Tbsp. peanut butter 1 C. cooked, dried beans or lentils					2	
FRUIT and VEGETABLES	Vitamin C rich: 4-6 oz. citrus juice 1 med. orange ½ grapefruit, cante-lope					1-2	
	Vitamin A. rich: ½ C. carrots, broc-coli, spinach, greens, sweet potatoes					1-2	
	Other: ½ C. potatoes peas, string beans, 1 med. apple, peach					1-2	
BREAD and CEREAL	1 slice enriched or whole grain bread 1 oz. (3/4 C.) dry cereal, 1/2 - 3/4 C. hot cereal Enriched noodles					3-4	
MISC.	Margarine, butter Desserts Sweets, candies						

COMMENTS:

2. Causes of a Vitamin A and Vitamin C deficiency would be lack of, or irregular consumption of, Vitamin A or C foods. Foods may have the vitamins, but they may be lost if improperly prepared. There may be poor liver storage of Vitamin A or absorption problems. Knowledge of nutrition might be lacking, or there might be insufficient funds. A practical solution would be a half-cup serving of orange juice per day or one medium orange, which supplies approximately 45 mg. of Vitamin C, the recommended allowance for adults. Inclusion of deep yellow and deep green fruits and vegetables or just an ounce of liver will supply about 4 to 5 thousand IU of Vitamin A, which is the minimal daily requirement. If you ate three ounces of liver, you would be having about 15,000 IU of Vitamin A stored for future use.

3. Certain things must be emphasized to all population groups. These include proper food handling, the sources of each nutrient, and reasons why each nutrient is vital. Supplementations, as well as knowledgeable food buying, will correct a deficiency.

4. Some patients state that the reason they avoid orange or grapefruit juice is that these juices give them stomach cramps so they switch to other beverages, like pure coffee. If they drink citrus juice either at the end or in the middle of the meal instead of at the beginning of the meal, they will not experience cramping. If there is difficulty in using foods that are natural sources of needed vitamins or minerals, then a multivitamin supplement should be taken daily with the physician's advice.

5. Constipation is common among the elderly. A cause could be reduced muscle tone or diminished activity. Practical solutions include increasing fluid intake to six or eight cups daily, a reasonable amount of exercise, and use of raw fruits and vegetables. If there is a problem chewing those raw fruits or vegetables, they can be chopped. Use whole wheat bread or bran in casseroles, meatloaf, and elsewhere to prevent constipation. Stewed prunes or figs are a traditional and effective aid to defecation. For some, applesauce is helpful.

Good diets are not necessarily costly, but more care and knowledge of food values are essential to remain adequately nourished on a limited list of inexpensive foodstuffs. Based on 1978 raw food cost in Roanoke, Virginia, breakfast meals cost about 30 to 40 cents, noon and night meals might cost 50 to 90 cents, averaging about $2.00 daily for balanced meals. This information is applicable in hospitals, extended care facilities, homes for adults or private homes. Nutrition is everyone's concern in all age groups.

Table 21.2. Cost analysis of economical foods
             meeting nutrient needs according to
             the basic 4 food groups

Breakfast	Raw food cost
4 oz. orange juice	.06
1 scrambled egg	.06
1 slice whole wheat toast	.04
1 t. margarine	.01
8 oz. milk	.11
8 oz. coffee	.03
	.31

Noon	
Sloppy Joes (1/2 C. on bun)	.20
1/2 C. carrott/raisin salad	.10
1/2 C. gelatin	.05
8 oz. milk	.11
Tea	.01
	.47

Night	
8 oz. Veg-Beef soup	.21
Peanut-butter/chopped prune sandwich	.18
Fresh fruit in season	.15
Decaffeinated coffee*	.04
	.58

*Recommended for those people who find that regu-
lar coffee give them problems sleeping at night.

Other tips for feeding the elderly include using plates
which are deep, as elderly persons frequently push food
against the sides of the plate to put it on the utensil.
Select proper size, weight, and contour of cups and glasses
to encourage adequate fluid intake. Many older people
prefer a lightweight mug to a cup and saucer.
   A word on therapeutic diets when indicated for the
elderly outpatient or long-term inpatient: Moderation rather
than restriction should be the rule of thumb. Individualize
the special diet so the older person can enjoy his prescribed
diet. Whenever nutrition counseling or diet therapy is
needed, consult your dietitian.

References

Nizel, Abraham E. "Role of Nutrition in the Oral Health
    of the Aging Patient." Dental Clinics of North
    America 20(3):569-584, 1976. Virginia Cooperative
    Extension Service. Foods for Older Folks. Publication
    243. Blacksburg, Va.: Virginia Polytechnic Institute
    and State University, 1977.
Robinson, Corinne H. "Nutrition in Later Maturity." In
    Fundamentals of Normal Nutrition, edited by Corinne H.
    Robinson. New York: Macmillan Publishing Co., 1978,
    pp. 328-335.

CHAPTER 22

DIETARY PLANNING

Janet M. Austin

This paper explores the role foods and liquids play as we
care for the elderly. Doctors, nurses, nursing assistants,
and other health care providers should be as aware of a
patient's nutritional needs as they are of medical assessment, nursing procedures, physical activities, and the like.
 How often is nutrition considered of primary importance
in treating the clinically ill? The first step in treatment
and prevention can be the presence of the dietitian at your
staff conferences, grand rounds, or ward rounds. Communication with this valuable team member should be as frequent
as it is with your M.D., head nurse, or other health professional. Invite dietitians to your staff conferences.
Consultations with your dietitian can be as important as a
surgical consultation concerning a gangrenous toe. They
will not only improve nutrition through better management
but will help you understand dietary causes and cures for
metabolic problems.
 When a nutritional assessment is needed, we are all
programmed to present past history, socioeconomic status,
physiological changes, and the presence of chronic disease.
How compulsive are we about our patient's nutrition?
Recently an 83-year-old man developed pneumonia that required
treatment on an acute medical service. After four weeks of
treatment, he returned to our unit with his mouth open, a
nasogastric tube in place, and cheeks and eyes were sunken.
All bony prominences were protruding. He had lost the ability
to speak, turn over in bed, or even scratch his own nose.
Somehow, his nutritional needs were overlooked. He had been
receiving a 400-calorie clear liquid diet for 4 weeks. A
serious oversight by his doctor! The x-rays, antibiotics
and chest physical therapy were conscientiously carried out.
But his nutrition was bypassed! This gentleman's nutrition
was restored, and today he is wheeling about in his wheelchair, feeding himself, and responding appropriately to
conversation.
 If you restore nutrition, support and follow-up on
rehabilitation, monitor medical problems, and provide per-
sonalized nursing care, you will have a body restored to a
quality of life. Poor nutrition leads to starved cells,
which are sick cells, abnormal in their function. The
result is mental, physical, and medical deterioration.
In a well-fed person the cells have oxygen plus food,
better metabolism, and a better functioning body, all due to
healthier cells. The patient has an increased ability to
be motivated and participate in therapy and rehabilitation.

In managing a patient's dietary regime, all facets must
be considered: medical problems, likes and dislikes, ability
to eat and drink, activity, normal value of nutrients, evaluation of laboratory data, status of disease, be it long-
term, short-term, or terminal. All of the above considerations should be included in developing treatment plans. Is
it always necessary to order low-salt diets or puree foods
for a patient with congestive heart failure or a patient
without teeth? Would you force fluids on a patient with
bone cancer that has metastasized to virtually every organ
in his body, simply because the medical books said a patient
should not die with a calcium level of 12.5. Surely you
would not insert a nasogastric tube or restrain this unfor-
tunate individual, who is pain-ridden, against his wishes.
As Dr. William Poe has stated, "The first lesson I learned
as a geriatrician was to protect my patients from doctoring."
     Have you really made an effort to make mealtime a
special time of day? Do your patients choose their menu?
Or have you accepted the routine food delivery without considering an individual's likes or dislikes? How long has it
been since you tested food for temperature or tasted it for
palatability? You may be amazed to find meat cold and ice
cream hot. Would you invite your family or boss to a sit-
down dinner, serving them from a tray from a delivery cart
for their reaction to the entree? If we were to change
places with our patients, we would improve service and look
for other methods besides unpalatable diets to provide treatment to our aged. The microwave oven is a great invention.
It would solve the problem of cold food and improve appetites.
It is our responsibility to approach those people who purchase
these items so that problems can be resolved. Managing
patients with congestive heart failure on diuretics, digitalis,
etc., may not be nearly as dangerous as a special diet that
results in malnutrition, weight loss, decreased activity,
pressure areas, pneumonia, and even death. If a patient is
eating poorly, be sure to evaluate all problems that may
cause anorexia. Did you give him horrid tasting potassium
chloride fizz? Did you give him phenothiazine concentrate
that leaves a wicked taste in one's mouth? Did you give him
nourishment heavy in consistency, one hour before lunch?
Did you give him drugs, such as digitalis, that are a known
appetite destroyer?
     Malnutrition, anorexia, and chronic brain syndromes often
lead our colleagues to nasogastric tube insertion as a routine
means of maintaining nutrition. Focus on comfort and quality
of life. If tubes are absolutely necessary, request the help
of your surgeon to insert a gastrostomy tube on those who
must be fed by other means. It is less offensive, more
comfortable, and reduces chance for aspiration. The importance of diet must be taught; it becomes as necessary to
eat food as it is to take Lasix, vitamins or stool softeners.
Time must be taken to feed our patients as conscientiously

as we would to bathe them or to change a sterile dressing.
Patience in feeding a patient may prevent many complications,
such as dehydration, pressure areas, or regression. Patients
should be taken to a dining room area that is cheerful and
pleasant. They should be sitting up and dressed up for the
occasion. Lying in bed in pajamas is hardly a setting for
dinner. For those patients who are terminally ill, meal
time may be the brightest hour during the day. Even if they
cannot swallow, allow them to fix their food, smell the
aroma, and enjoy the service. Families and friends should
be encouraged to bring home-cooked foods, provided your staff
has helped them to understand the restrictions or special
needs of the patient. Recently we encouraged our volunteers
to hold a potluck dinner for our long-term hospitalized
veterans, so they could have some home-cooked foods and the
privilege of choice. Make changes and bend rules that are
often made for our benefit and not our patients. We go home
after eight hours, they often remain for months and even
years.

     In summary, consider a nutritional assessment a priority
in developing your patient's treatment plan. Don't sideline
your dietitians; they are most valuable. Use your skills
and knowledge to promote health through sensible diet,
treatment, and management. If you educate your patient,
families, and staff, you will create an acute awareness of
nutritional needs and provide methods to maintain diet without undue stress to your patient.

CHAPTER 23

DISEASES AND TREATMENTS AFFECTING NUTRITION IN THE ELDERLY

A. Sidney Barritt

This paper will examine some diseases and some treatments affecting nutrition in the elderly.

What happens to the gut as it gets older? Does it work as well as it does in youth and middle age? In some ways, it does not. For instance, acid secretion falls with age and pancreatic secretion of enzymes may also fall. Does this make any difference? Acid secretion is not absolutely critical to assimilation of food, and as there is so much reserve pancreatic secretion that this usually isn't a problem unless there is pancreatic disease. Motor function declines as one gets older or, put another way, the transit time of food from one end of the gastrointestinal tract to the other slows down. This has nothing to do with assimilation of food, but change in motor function gives rise to symptoms: indigestion in one end of the tract and constipation at the other. These symptoms lead to changes in attitudes toward food in general and for foods in particular if their intake is reliably associated with these symptoms. These changes in the aging gut don't affect its ability to absorb nutrients. Preliminary data suggest that occasionally some forms of dietary folic acid are not well absorbed, but there is little difference in the ability of the gut of the older person to absorb other nutrients.

What are some problems that will impinge on nutrition? Surgery causes nutritional problems although most are short-term. Long-term problems are apt to occur when surgery involves the gastrointestinal tract. When one is operated on for ulcer disease, the vagus nerve which controls acid secretion and, to a lesser degree, other secretions in the gut is cut and usually part of the stomach is taken out. This works pretty well. It cures ulcers and ulcers rarely recur. Long-term nutritional consequences not obvious in the immediate follow-up period ought to be considered. In a series of patients who were followed for 20 years, 20% lost more than 5% of their preoperative weight. Some reasons are that the amount of stomach left is smaller, and after this operation persons can no longer tolerate the same volume of food at a meal (1). Dietary habits change. The operation also induces a subtle form of malabsorption. The vagus nerve controls release a number of secretions throughout the gut. These are exquisitely timed to coincide with the arrival of food. This not only refers to acid secretion of the stomach but also to biliary secretions by the gallbladder and pancreatic enzyme secretion by the pancreas. When this exquisite timing is lost, malabsorption, particularly of fat, results and there is weight loss. Another consequence of malabsorption of fat affects one's bone density. When fat

is malabsorbed, Vitamin D and calcium are also malabsorbed. Although not
a problem in short-term follow-ups, 20-year follow-up
studies suggest that about 25%-30% of people will have bone
disease consequent to ulcer surgery if they are followed
long enough (2). With regard to Vitamin D and calcium
absorption, the abnormality may not be a problem to a
middle-aged adult, but it is vitally important because it
coincides with osteoporosis 15-20 years later in the older
adult.

Anemia is a problem. If people are followed 15-20
years, as many as 40% become iron deficient and thereby
anemic. Vitamin B12 losses account for 10%-15% becoming
deficient (3). What was a suitable operation in youth and
middle-age may have disastrous nutritional consequences
when the patient is seen 20 to 30 years later.

Intestinal bypass is done for forms of obesity that
can't be controlled with any form of dietary regimen. We
do not know what is going to happen to these patients 15-20
years later. The operation deliberately excludes most of
the small intestine, where absorption occurs from the food
stream, and deliberately induces malabsorption. This is
fine for an obese person who weighs 400 pounds and who has
very successfully adapted to weighing 200 pounds in youth
and early middle-age. What will happen to them in older
age? Nobody knows. We need to follow them to anticipate
problems or to prevent their occurrence.

Cancer surgery is a large topic and it is difficult to
include everything about it. When part of the intestinal
tract has been removed or bypassed, some obvious things can
be done to prevent the occurrence of nutritional deficiency.
A tube can be placed or a special diet can be fabricated
to take the part of the removed part of the intestinal
tract. These problems are obvious and anticipation should
be simple. The nonspecific problems that are hard to pinpoint are changes in appetite toward eating in the cancer
patient. There are no pat answers.

Some therapies which we use can be a cause of malabsorption. Considering the gallons of antacids swigged or
the bushels of tablets taken, antacids are useful and safe
drugs. We rarely appreciate the complications. The absorption of phosphorus is inhibited by certain antacids, particularly aluminum ones. This can lead to a low level of
phosphorus in the blood, which leads to osteomalacia, defec-
tive calcification of the bone matrix. With regard to
calcium and Vitamin D metabolism, when this coincides with
osteoporosis, which may be a natural process of aging, the
result can be catastrophic. Another problem may be phos-
phorus-depletion syndrome, which is hard to characterize
because it presents, with poor appetite, a sense of malaise
and easy fatigability. It occurs rarely but is amenable
to easy treatment by either the addition of phosphorus or
reduction in the amount of antacids. Aluminum-containing

antacids inhibit Vitamin A absorption. Vitamin A is
necessary for optimal vision. Magnesium-containing
antacids induce diarrhea and, by definition, malabsorption
of fluid and electrolytes. Certain antacids also inhibit
iron absorption. With drug interactions, antacids may
bind antibiotics that are simultaneously administered,
rendering antibiotics ineffective. Tetracycline is the
one we know most about.

The effects of alcohol are widespread and are certainly not confined to the elderly. The spectrum of the
effects of alcohol abuse may be different in one group as
opposed to another. Some people are exquisitely sensitive
to the effects of alcohol on the stomach. Alcohol induces
both chronic and acute inflammation, which results in
nausea and loss of appetite. The small bowel mucosa is
altered. This is where most absorption occurs and so
malabsorption is a problem, particularly that of folate.
Folate is necessary for normal formation of red blood cells.
In turn, folic acid deficiency causes further malabsorption
leading to a vicious cycle. The secretions of biliary and
pancreatic ducts and glands are needed for absorption of
fat. Alcohol damages the liver, altering the amount of
bile that can be made. It can also damage the pancreas,
altering the amount of enzymes which can be made. So
damage to either of these organs is potentially deleterious
to nutrition.

A bowel movement a day is not necessary to good health
despite what some believe. The corollary to that belief
is that you need to take a laxative if you don't have a
good bowel movement every day. Often that is not a problem:
all it involves is being dependent on a cathartic or enema.
In some people this leads to loss of protein from the gut,
a problem for an older person rather than for a younger
person. This habit can lead to malabsorption of fat. Both
can be severe nutritional problems. Agents involved in
causing this kind of malnutrition are usually the irritative
types of laxatives such as phenolphthalein, bisacodyl,
oxyphenisatin and cascara, which are in a number of
preparations.

Cholestyramine is not a commonly used drug but it has
been used to control cholesterol levels. It binds
cholesterol as well as bile salts. By binding bile salts
it interferes with fat absorption and causes malnutrition.
By interfering with fat absorption, it interferes with
absorption of fat-soluble vitamins--A, D, and K. Cholestyramine also binds digitalis-type drugs and thus may render
the concomitant use of digitalis ineffective.

Congestive heart failure is a common problem in the
aged, but its nutritional complications are rarely considered.
Anorexia, or poor appetite, is a vague symptom with many
potential causes. In congestive heart failure, the failing

heart allows blood to back up through the intertinal tract and this leads to sensations of indigestion and poor appetite Paradoxically, we use digitalis to improve contractions of a failing heart and a toxic effect of digitalis is anorexia. Therefore, it may be difficult in the clinical setting to determine whether this patient's poor appetite is due to congestive heart failure or a change in his digitalis prescription.

Retention of salt and, ultimately, water is the body's response to congestive heart failure. This leads to fluid accumulation, so we attack this by restricting the amount of salt in the diet. This restricts dietary choices and, for some people, makes the diet absolutely unpalatable and unacceptable.

Dyspnea. If one is really short of breath on account of congestion of the lungs, it may be difficult to enjoy eating or just to eat. Finally, the same process causing atherosclerosis also affects blood vessels that serve the intestine and this may cause pain during meals, loss of the mucus membrane lining of the intestine, and, thereby, malabsorption. Again, we use digitalis as a treatment and digitalis decreases the amount of blood flow that gets to the intestine and so may exacerbate the problem, leading to a real clinical dilemma.

This is a brief and less than inclusive outline of a number of medical and therapeutic problems affecting nutrition. The problems are not absolutely specific to elderly persons, but they are certainly more common and are less well tolerated. The examples cited need therapeutic intervention but, more importantly, anticipation to prevent their occurrence in the first place.

References

(1) Pryor, J. P., M. J. O'Shea, P. L. Brooks, and G. K. Datar. "The Long-Term Metabolic Consequences of Partial Gastrectomy." Am. J. Med. 51:5-10, 1971.

(2) Eddy, Richard L. "Metabolic Bone Disease after Gastrectomy." Am. J. Med. 50:442-449, 1971.

(3) Pryor. "Consequences of Partial Gastrectomy."

Part V

Specific Medical Problems of the Elderly

INTRODUCTION

Harold B. Haley

These papers are definitive monographs covering the current
status of major aspects of common health problems.

James Folsom, a pioneer in caring for the mental
problems of the elderly, describes the history and current
status of reality orientation and attitude therapy. He
presents different applications of these approaches to the
needs of individual patients. He discusses the medical
literature analyses of reality orientation, both in terms
of critics and rebuttals to the critics. Currently, he is
developing a day treatment center for elderly patients.

James Bryan thinks through the nature and etiology of
cancer and demographic data and mortality relating to
elderly patients. He analyzes the effects of diagnostic
procedures on patients--discomfort, cost, time--making a
cost-benefit analysis of these procedures on patients.

Three papers on urinary tract disease are presented.
Ralph Goldman details changes in renal anatomy and loss of
physiological function of the kidney which occurs with age.

Charles Schleupner has written a definitive paper on
urinary infection in the elderly. Complete discussion is
made of epidemiology, bacteriuria, pathogenesis, pathophysiology, etiologic agents of infection and are described with
emphasis on diagnosis and treatment of acute cystitis,
pyelonephritis, and catheter-associated infections.

Jorge Roman gives an overview of end-stage renal disease
in the elderly and the various places in treatment of diet,
hemo- and peritoneal dialysis, drugs, and kidney transplants.

An important medical problem involving all diseases and
all therapeutic approaches is that of prescribing drugs.
Richard Lindsay analyzes the demography of prescribing drug-
prescribing, induced diseases, physiological changes due to aging
and their effects on drug action, the "anti-cholinergic syndrome,"
and preventing drug toxicity.

This part closes with a paper describing how a distinguished physician, Dr. Eugene Stead, and his distinguished
patients interact and improve the quality of living of
each. It should be read by every medical student and every
physician.

CHAPTER 24

DEVELOPMENT AND UTILIZATION OF
ATTITUDE THERAPY AND REALITY ORIENTATION

James C. Folsom

Overview

For ideal care of the elderly this paper considers positive
effects of utilizing reality orientation, attitude therapy,
and a treatment team approach with involvement of both
ancillary staff and their clients.

Pilot programs and papers concerning use and abuse of
reality orientation are reviewed. Reality orientation is
treated as an ongoing process involving the environmental
reality of the client. Day Center treatment and the importance of a supportive social setting is discussed. The
major theme presented is that dementia in the aged can be
correctable, even cured.

Historical Considerations

In late 1950 Dr. Folsom represented Topeka Veterans
Administration Hospital on the rehabilitation subcommittee
of the Governor's Committee of the White House Conference
on Aging. Meanwhile, the Veterans Administration (V.A.)
Central Office became concerned about projections of numbers
of elderly veteran patients for 1970s and 1980s.

Few programs in the V.A. system held much hope of
helping solve problems of the elderly. Once those dreaded
labels "senility," "senile dementia," "chronic brain
syndrome," "organic brain syndrome," "cerebral arteriosclerosis," "Alzheimer's Disease," or "Pick's Disease" were
applied to an individual, it was downhill all the way to the
nursing home (or State Hospital for Insane) and then a
merciful death.

At Topeka V.A. Hospital we established a 50-bed
Rehabilitation Bed Service for geriatric mental patients
and began a pilot study using full-treatment potential of
all employees.

A reevaluation of patient care indicated that patients'
physical needs were being met, but emotional needs required
attention. Nursing assistants were given time to visit and
learn treatment objectives of other units. Regular meetings
of nursing assistants with the nursing supervisor were begun
and later replaced by meetings with a full rehabilitation
team. Importance of nursing assistants as team members was
stressed and their initiative in creating activity programs
was encouraged (1).

Before the new program began, 50 elderly psychiatric
patients were living on the ward with intensive nursing

attention. They were allowed to do almost nothing for fear
they might fall and hurt themselves. During the day the
50 patients sat in air-conditioned comfort in a beautiful
new dayroom--staring off into space, mumbling to themselves,
ignoring everything that went on around them, expecting and
getting total care and having no responsibilities other than
to breathe, swallow, and excrete (at times even the latter
two functions were handled for them by gavage or enema tubes
and catheters). Fourteen of these patients spent most of
their time in wheelchairs. Injury rate and recurrent illness
rate was high. Hospital employees shunned this ward and had
to be forced to accept tours of duty. Time off for sickness
and accidents was high.

A few months of intensive rehabilitation team care
altered the picture. Careful review of records of 14
patients confined to wheelchairs revealed no clear-cut
reason for their use. Physical therapy, together with the
new care-for-yourself attitude, enabled 10 patients to
permanently leave their wheelchairs. Small group activities
focused on involving patients with the environment and with
other human beings.

Soon an air of liveliness pervaded the unit. Patients
and personnel were anxious to complete daily toileting and
ward housekeeping duties so they could get on with more
interesting activities. Each patient was screened to
determine his fullest potential. Instead of sitting around
the dayroom staring carefully over the heads of their fellow
inmates, patients began conversing and making friends.

Activity areas sprang up on the ward. The visiting room
was converted into a workshop for occupational therapy and
ceramics. Industrial therapy assignments were arranged for
the more able-bodied. A grounds detail was quite successful
and, when colder weather arrived, projects had to be found
inside because many of the men insisted on getting away from
the ward part of every day. The ward personnel supported
the patients wholeheartedly.

There was a decrease in employee lost-time accidents
and use of sick leave. Patients had fewer injuries and
recurrent infections. Attitudes of employees toward the
geriatric patients changed. Instead of shunning this unit,
there was a waiting list of personnel who wanted to transfer
to this unit. Having a group of employees who enjoyed
working together was most gratifying. Improvement in the
entire ward situation and in individual patients was worth
the effort.

Before the Aide Centered Activity Program for Elderly
Patients, there was little communication among ward staff
members. To improve communication skills and develop a
treatment program, concepts of attitude therapy were taught.

Attitude Therapy and Reality Orientation

Attitude therapy is a communication tool that promotes
development of a therapeutic environment--a definite
therapeutic structuring or shaping of environment. Mallory
et al. felt that a treatment-centered milieu offers each
patient corrective living and learning experiences and,
regardless of the patient's diagnosis, he can learn better
ways of relating to others (2). Folsom considers attitude
therapy a communication device (3). It communicates
feelings, knowledge, and a therapeutic approach to staff
persons in order to give them a better understanding of
therapeutic potential and needs of the patient.

Therefore, attitude therapy enables staff members to
become more client-oriented, as well as more aware of their
own skills and attributes. All staff levels are encouraged
to communicate in an effective problem-solving setting.
They are communicating, not only verbally, but also on a
behavioral level. A nursing assistant is no longer a "human
janitor" but an integral member of the treatment team.
Everyone coming in contact with the patient is involved in
planning and shares in the responsibility of carrying out
treatment goals. The staff must feel capable, (i.e., well),
if the client is to recover.

Attitude therapy had its beginnings at the Menninger
Foundation in Topeka, Kansas, from 1925 to 1935. A 1950
revision of the Foundation's "Guide to the Order Sheet"
formulated the theory that, for the system of patient treatment to work, everyone with whom the patient came in contact
must maintain the same general attitude toward him. How we
say things and the atmosphere created through our attitudes
is more important than what we say and what we do. Patients
react to our feelings and our manner more than they do to
our words (4). Formation of a treatment team using attitude
therapy as its communication device and therapeutic approach
helps to achieve consistency in all its contacts with the
patient. Thus, the staff has a shorthand method of conveying
a great deal of information concerning the patient. In
addition, concepts of attitude therapy are easily learned
and can be communicated rapidly and clearly from one person
to another. The five basic attitudes are: active friendliness, passive friendliness, kind firmness, matter-of-fact,
and no demand (5). One of the above attitudes is selected
in treating the patient, and followed through evaluation of
the patient's psychopathology. Consistency in approach is
of paramount importance.

As staff modify their own inappropriate behaviors toward
a client who is exhibiting maladaptive behavior, they realize
the client can also relearn behavior. In a reality-oriented
hospital, maladaptive behavior is no longer rewarded or
expected (6). The hospital environment becomes such that a

client is seen as a person capable of relearning adaptive
behavior. In turn, staff members become more aware of their
roles in planning and implementing treatment goals. In
essence, these programs are for staff first and for client
second. If the staff is not oriented and motivated, neither
will the client be.

In 1960 another attitude therapy program was initiated
at the Mental Health Institute in Mt. Pleasant, Iowa. Dr.
Lerner, a staff internist, decided to use methods he had
observed in treatment of acute mental patients in handling
hospitalized geriatric cases. Only 3% of geriatric patients
had improved enough to return to prehospital adjustment
despite staff work. Staff members interested in working on
a pilot project with geriatric cases were recruited. The
idea was to utilize available personnel to the fullest extent
and to emphasize various techniques of attitude therapy. To
be admitted to this new pilot study geriatric ward, patients
had to be over 65, able to walk, a new admission, and mentally
ill. Degree of illness, such as total disorientation,
incontinence of urine and feces, smearing of excreta, etc.,
was no bar to admission to the program.

Staff were encouraged to keep treatment philosophies
as simple as possible and to keep their thinking uncluttered
as possible by omitting the usual psychiatric jargon and
medical diagnoses. Within six months the staff had established guidelines and developed techniques for helping the
confused elderly patient reorient himself to reality.

On admission, careful orientation to the ward was considered of utmost importance, even though the patient
exhibited no evidence of being aware of what was going on.
A baseline of acceptance, concern, and expectation of
participation in one's own recovery was established. A
feeling of calmness, consistency, and security was communicated to the patient. He could now give up some of his
feelings of loneliness, worthlessness, apathy, confusion,
and disorientation. The staff was trying to help him to
give up his illness.

Each patient was considered carefully to find areas of
"wellness." When such an area was found, efforts were made
to expand its boundaries. Of utmost importance was keeping
the ward environment as calm as possible, reinforcing the
staff's valiant efforts to remain calm despite any disturbance, thereby encouraging patients to do likewise.

At first, some patients seemed to know nothing, not
even their own name. With such patients the staff made
repeated efforts throughout day and night to call the
patient's attention to his own name and help him to relearn
who he was. The patient was encouraged to accept the fact
that he was in a mental hospital and the treatment team held
out hope for his eventual return to his own community living.

When the pilot study was presented, the team joined in writing guidelines, the essence of the program. The program was called reality orientation when guidelines were written in 1962, as follows:

Reality Orientation, as we use it, implies a specific set of ideas to be followed. They are:
1. A calm environment.
2. A set routine.
3. Clear responses to patients' questions, and the same types of questions should be asked of the patient.
4. Talk clearly to the patient, not necessarily loud.
5. Direct patients around by clear directions. If need be, guide them to and from their destinations.
6. Remind them of the date, time, etc.
7. Don't let them stay confused by allowing them to ramble in their speech, actions, etc.
8. Be firm as necessary.
9. Be sincere.

Two years later the chief nurse added: "Make requests of patients in a calm manner, implying the patient will comply," and "consistency."

After six months of pilot study, "Reality Orientation for the Elderly Mental Patient," 49% of patients admitted improved sufficiently to return to their prehospital adjustment. After one year, 57% of the patients returned to their prehospital adjustment.

In January 1965 a program of reality orientation (R.O.) was started on a geriatric ward at the Tuscaloosa V.A. Hospital (7). The purpose of the program was to practice reality orientation 24 hours a day for these psychiatric, medically infirm patients. Orientation to reality is taken at its most basic meaning. If the patient does not know his own name, he is taught. If he does not know where he is and where he is from, he is told. Then he is taught such things as the day, week, month, year, and his age.

Reorientation to reality goes on around the clock. The patient is constantly reminded of who he is, where he is, why he is there, and what we expect. In addition, there are specific classes in reorientation. These are divided into two parts--a basic class meeting one-half hour twice a day, seven days a week, and an advanced classes meeting once a day Monday through Friday.

The R.O. classrooms, reality boards, and other props are adjunctive to 24-hour-a-day concentration of staff in every contact with the patient on current reality. Without the 24-hour-a-day program, basic and advanced R.O. classes are worthless and can be harmful. Imagine the shock experienced by a professional visiting a nursing home that claimed to be using R.O. techniques when he observed patients tied in their chairs, babbling incoherently. He asked the

nurse about the R.O. program, only to be told, "They have
all graduated." R.O. is a process, not a thing represented
by classroom instruction and reality boards.

As the reality orientation program for elderly mental
patients was developing, the same techniques were used in
treating younger patients with severe brain damage. Staff
were impressed with results in these cases.

Reality orientation may be defined as follows: Reality
orientation (R.O.) is a technique designed to return to the
confused person the maximum use of his assets. It rests
on the belief that no one is totally and permanently confused.
R.O. is a process in which family members, staff persons,
and the clients themselves, talk about what is actually
happening in the here and now--one's name, name of companion,
weather, day of week, date, room, furniture, expectation of
a meal. Reality as it is understood in R.O. is related to
person (self-identity, identity of others); place (awareness
of surroundings); and time (awareness of past, present, and
future).

Basically, R.O. is a person-to-person technique that
involves anyone who comes into contact with the confused
person. Some overall concepts are included in the following
statements:

1. In every person, regardless of illness or infirmity
there is a sphere of well-being, of nonconfusion, that must
be worked with.

2. Clients are people to be treated as individuals. As
people they assume responsibility for their own rehabilitation (return to reality) as soon as possible.

3. Clients, as people, need to know what is expected
of them and what they can expect of others.

4. The client's environment, including family, friends,
and staff, must continuously reinforce reality--identity,
time and place.

5. Factors that might contribute to the client's
disorientation should be investigated and, if possible,
remedied.

6. Treatment must always be based on client
involvement.

Modification of client's inappropriate behavior must
be promoted by appropriate behavior on the part of family
members and staff persons. This emphatic approach uses
five attitudes or approaches reinforcing adult-to-adult
behavior. They also provide a guide for appropriate behavior
by staff and family when the client is "acting out" and
confused.

Individual differences, such as knowledge of past life-
style, attitudes, ethnic background, social life space, and
medical history must be considered holistically as part of
total autonomous reality and personality makeup.

     Assessment of a client must include, not only his
recall and retention, but his ability to function more
effectively within his environment. Remember, reality
orientation is not a cure-all. Its long-range effects
may include increased social interaction, increased
independence in activities of daily living, and greater
awareness of others in the environment.
     Successful reality orientation programs promote self-
respect and self-sufficiency. Concepts inherent in a therapeutic community setting are important elements in
reorientation. Through restructured environment, provision
of more audiovisual aids, and work of an informed staff,
the client is motivated continuously in an adult-to-adult
manner to maintain contact with other people, places, and
time elements. Systematic review of essential elements of
reality (identity, time and place), stimulates unused
neurological pathways. This helps the client to develop
new ways of functioning or to resume former successful
transactions (8).
     Reality orientation has been criticized on several
occasions in recent literature. Gubrium and Ksander
reported on what was a caricature of reality orientation
and it is obvious the staff person needed orientation
more than the patients (9).
     With regard to organic brain syndrome, Dr. Wershow
suggested that "we abandon our fantasies of therapeutic
omnipotence, that we cease the terribly expensive and
useless therapies vigorously conducted over long periods
which always turn out to be no more than minimal in their
effect" (10). Wershow's article drew response. Dr. Settin
pointed out that 12.5% of a randomly selected group of
subjects presenting an organic brain syndrome were found to
be suffering from potentially treatable diseases. There is
a striking percentage of elderly doomed to eventual
"functioning at no more than a vegetative level" (as Wershow
stated), for lack of treatment. Settin concludes: "As
clinicians, we cannot disregard our responsibility to the
small but not insignificant proportion of aging persons who
are being erroneously labeled as irreversibly senile. Until
further research rules out (1) the use of the term 'senility'
in favor of more explicit diagnostic labels, and (2) the
use of the term 'Organic Brain Syndrome' for reversible
conditions, the current and future status of Organic Brain
Syndrome statistics will remain an unknown quantity" (11).
     Dr. Cohen takes issue with Wershow's statement that
organic brain syndrome "is inexorably progressive, that it
progresses from increasing cognitive and judgmental
disability to eventual (if death does not intervene)
complete helplessness, total dependency, loss of sphincter
control, in short, functioning at no more than a vegetative

level." Cohen states, "OBS can also be caused by trauma,
infection, vascular disease, metabolic disease, tumor,
etc., and need not be deteriorating or even irreversible.
OBS patients can deteriorate; some can deteriorate, then
stabilize; some have a non-progressive disorder; some have
a disorder of varying degrees of reversibility" (12).

Dr Armstrong responds to Wershow by saying that nursing
care should be oriented toward helping the patient with
organic brain damage to live as fully as possible rather
than simply to "make him comfortable" until he dies.

Armstrong stresses the fact that through in-service
training information has been passed along to lesser-paid
staff who have day-to-day personal contact with the patients.
"The technical skills . . . are basically common sense and
honesty. The quality of caring does not come with years
of schooling, degrees, or price. . . . it can be developed
in all but the very callous or the very uncaring, and,
alas, in highly trained specialists who are committed to
the theory that unproductive people and people who won't get
well aren't worth their time and attention" (13).

Wershow asks that we attend to the needs of less-
trained aides, LPN's and others "who bear the brunt of
caring for these patients, surely one of the least rewarding
jobs imaginable." We are in complete agreement with him
that this is very often the case. Indeed, that is what
reality orientation is all about. Its beginning was "An
Aide Centered Program for Elderly Patients." The basic
concept is that those less trained staff members (LPN's,
nurses' aides, food service workers, and housekeeping aides),
who are with the patient the most, must have adequate
supervision and emotional support if they are to be
participants in reality orientation. Dr. Armstrong's reply
regarding the demands a therapeutic program places on staff:
"What it does demand is staff who are committed to the
principle that human life is precious at every age; who are
sensitive to the needs, spoken and unspoken, of other
persons; who respect people because they are human, and
who lay as few stereotypes as possible on the people with
whom they work" (14).

Day Treatment Centers

In January 1978 we opened a day center for elderly persons
living in the community who were experiencing confusion,
disorientation, and memory loss.

The program utilizes reality orientation, attitude
therapy and team approach. Family members and elderly
participants are members of the treatment team.

A therapeutic program is designed for elderly persons
who are experiencing mild to severe degrees of confusion
and disorientation. Emphasis is placed on improving

functional capacities for better personal hygiene,
relearning housekeeping skills, ability to utilize public
transportation, and community services.

In addition, resocialization and community activities
are offered to increase the sense of personal worth, life
experiences, and social relationships. Our primary objective
is to enable participants to remain in the community by
providing rehabilitative services for older persons and
their families.

I.C.D. makes available its full service, education, and
research resources to the program. Specific services
include: social adjustment services; physical health services, including physical therapy and occupational therapy;
vocational and industrial rehabilitation services; speech
and hearing services; activities of daily living retraining;
therapeutic recreational activities; nutritional midday
meal; and multidisciplinary team evaluations.

The center is in operation three days a week from
9:30 a.m. to 2:30 p.m. Basic concepts remain the same,
however, and the validity of reality orientation is being
affirmed again. Our experience to date is both fascinating
and encouraging.

The story of Mr A. is a good illustration.

Mr. A came with his daughter for the initial interview.
He had gotten lost that morning trying to find her apartment
and he arrived looking tense and, although fully dressed,
had a "not together" overall appearance and manner.

Mr. A is a tall, outdoor-type man, 63-years old, who
was widowed four months before the interview. The family
became aware of loss of memory four years ago. He had full
medical work-ups in 1974 and December 1977. Diagnoses
included: presenile dementia, Alzheimer's disease and
cerebral arteriosclerosis.

Formerly a near genius with mechanical things, he had
lost all mechanical ability--couldn't dial a phone, get
zippers to work, or get keys to open doors. Early in the
program he was continually confused--coming at wrong times
and on wrong days. In the program he was constantly losing
his newspaper, hat, and coat. Orientation therapy evaluation
showed glaring deficiencies.

He was given a pocket calendar and he learned to use it
and not lose it. We helped him deal with his anxieties,
his widowhood, and other traumatic losses. In intensive
counseling he was helped to reorganize his daily activities.
He decided he had always moved too fast, had always done
too many things at once, often thinking about what he was
going to do next instead of what he was presently doing.
He told us he needed to slow down and pay attention to
what he was doing.

Within two months he was renewing old friendships and
stated that he wanted to practice math--work on addition,

subtraction, multiplication and division--and dialing a
telephone. After three months in the program, Mr. A
asked a counselor, "When do people around here realize
that a person does not need any more instructions?"

After four months he was able to leave the program.
A letter from Mr. A following his self-discharge was
coherent and well put. He was caring for his sister's
apartment, flowers, and dog while she was in the hospital.
A later phone conversation indicated he was still at his
sister's helping her following her hospitalization.

Within a few months, Mr. A's ability to function
deteriorated again as he became more anxious and disorgan-
ized. His basic need for his own place to live was unmet.

His daughter helped him arrange for a studio apartment
in an adult residence. The complex has a drugstore, tavern,
gift shop, delicatessen, post office, bank, and indoor
swimming pool. There are lounges, craft and game rooms, a
full activity schedule, and three meals are served in the
dining room.

The first few weeks were stormy. His children, sisters,
and other relatives visited him often. Then one night he
"had a terrific time at a dance." One lady in particular
"was quite a looker."

Suddenly his little apartment was very nice, the food
great and the people friendly. For now Mr. A is doing well.
How much of his dysfunction was and is due to Alzheimer's
disease? Will his functional capacity continue to improve
in a setting where his basic needs for a home and close
personal relationships are met? Specific answers to these
questions lie in the future. We think Mr. A would tell you
that right now today is sufficient unto itself.

This case illustrates the major philosophy of reality
orientation--to engage an individual in a reality that is
meaningful, that life has a continuum despite age or
infirmity. Mr. A's need, beyond assistance with reorganizing
day-to-day activities, was need for love and recognition as a
man capable of meaningful activities.

We welcome "hopeless cases" in the Center for Developmental Aging. They are far and away the most fascinating
patients one could have. Their improvement also brings the
greatest satisfaction to staff.

The treatment program is challenging because causes of
dementia are so varied and each individual is unique.

We work with patient, relatives, and ourselves, and
we all change in the process. Every confused and disoriented
older person who comes through our door is treated as a case
of correctable dementia. Our shared challenge is to bring
that about.

References

(1)   Brown, E. L. Newer Dimensions of Patient Care, Part
      II. New York: Russell Sage Foundation, 1962.
(2)   Mallory, J., D. Murphy, and H. Coppedge. "An Attitude
      Therapy Program in a Teaching Hospital." Hospital and
      Community Psychiatry 20(4) 99-102, 1969.
(3)   Folsom, J. C. "Attitude Therapy as a Communication
      Device." Transactions 1, 18-21, 1969.
(4)   The Menninger Foundation. Guide to the Order Sheet
      (Revised. 4-195, M. F.-188). Unpublished Manuscript,
      1950.
(5)   "The Treatment Team: Attitude Therapy and the Team
      Approach." Mental Hospitals 16:307-320, 1965.
(6)   Taulbee, E. E., and J. C. Folsom. "Attitude Therapy:
      A Behavior Therapy Approach," in R. M. Jurjevich (ed.),
      Direct Psychotherapy: 28 American Originals, 1, Coral
      Gables, Florida: University of Miami Press. 1973,
      pp. 169-189.
(7)   Taulbee, L. R., and J. C. Folsom. "Reality Orientation
      for Geriatric Patients." Hospital and Community
      Psychiatry 17:133-135, 1966.
(8)   Stephens, L. P., J. C. Folsom, and L. R. Taulbee.
      "Introduction to Reality Orientation." Reality Orienta-
      tion, Washington, D.C.: American Psychiatric Association,
      1975.
(9)   Gubrium, J. F., and M. Ksander. "On Multiple Realities
      and Reality Orientation." Gerontologist 15:142-145,
      1975.
(10) Wershow, H. J. "Comment: Reality Orientation for
      Gerontologists, Some Thoughts about Senility."
      Gerontologist 17 (4):297-302, 1977.
(11) Settin, J. M. "Comment: Some Thoughts about Diseases
      Presenting as Senility." Gerontologist 18 (1):71-72,
      1978.
(12) Cohen, G. D. "Comment: Organic Brain Syndrome, Reality
      Orientation for Critics of Clinical Interventions."
      Gerontologist 18 (3):313-314, 1978.
(13) Armstrong, P. W. "Comment: More Thoughts on Senility."
      Gerontologist 18 (3):315-316, 1978.
(14) Ibid., p. 316.

CHAPTER 25

CANCER IN THE ELDERLY

James A. Bryan II

In primitive societies if the "true" name of a person or
object was known, you had the power over that particular
thing. In more modern times Bacon stated that the first
step toward scientifically understanding anything was to
name and define it so that common observations could be
shared. This paper is about cancer, but the name "cancer"
alone gives me neither power, insight nor greater capability
to do good for my patients; hence it must not be a "true"
name. Nevertheless, it is a start in trying to cope with a
common occurrence usually linked with death, destruction,
and biological violence.
    We want to come to grips with the name "cancer" and
its associated problems as it occurs and affects older folk.
We will review incidence, prevalence, and age-specific
occurrence, as well as current approaches and costs of
caring for cancer patients, along with consideration of life
values reflected in choices of care made.

Occurrence

Cancer occurs at all ages, in all races, in both sexes, in
all parts of the country, in all parts of the body and in
all variations of biologic behavior. Why is cancer so much
a part of old age and why does it carry such mortal
connotations?
    Several observations and definitions need to be made:
    1. Cancer is a broad term applied to the malignant
proliferation of a cell of a particular tissue origin that
is usually more or less responsive to normal cellular growth
control mechanisms. Cancer causes illness and death by its
local growth and/or spread to more distant sites with
interference with normal bodily functions.
    2. Cancer generally occurs with increasing frequency
with increasing age. From an epidemiologic point of view
this can be interpreted as (a) those who are going to have
cancer have favorable biological characteristics that
enable them to live long enough to have cancer or (b), more
likely, if you live long enough you have a chance of one or
more of your cells yielding to the cancer causing influences
that accumulate. This is an attractive idea, because studies
link certain cancers with certain chronic effectors such as
tar, cigarettes, radiation, certain drugs, asbestos, actinic
radiation, hormonal imbalances, etc. Some of this would be
reflected in the cancer types dependent on occupational or
environmental exposures. This would support some ideas

about environmental differences accounting for the
differing rates of cancer in different parts of the country
or between countries. (Cancer death rate runs parallel with
degree of industrialization.)
     3. Cancer in any individual is the summation of a
number of forces which have been acting over time. One
model which has been drawn has included the vectors of
socioenvironmental, behavioral, and biological influences
within a person of a particular genetic background. The
only problem with this model is it doesn't account for the
time axis, or the body's capacity to correct and control
aberrant phenomenon in its cells. Can we use such observations as cancer case clustering in families, communities, or
industries; racial variations in cancer patterns; or cancer
associations with dietary habits (either positively or
negatively such as sugar or roughage) to gain any insight?
     Table 25.1 shows the death rates for malignant neo-
plasms of digestive origin in the United States.

Table 25.1. Death rates for gastrointestinal malignancies

All ages	49/100,000
10	0.2
25 - 34	2.4
35 - 44	11.0
45 - 54	43.0
55 - 64	121.0
65 - 74	267.0
75 - 84	450.0
85	660.0

The chance of dying from a gastrointestinal malignancy is
increasing with time in this country. This death rate table
does not reflect the approximately 50% success rate in
dealing with these cancers.
     Table 25.2 shows another common type of cancer (1) with
a little different pattern of expression.

Table 25.2. Death rates for respiratory malignancies

All ages	Male - 43/100,000	Female - 8/100,000	Both sexes
35 - 44	13	4	25/1,000,000
45 - 54	59	13	
55 - 64	162	21	
65 - 74	263	30	
75 - 84	221	39	
85	161	49	

Here males clearly predominate and the peak incidence occurs in the 65-74 age group; this rate included the 90,000+ lung cancer deaths, 8,000+ deaths from cancer of the mouth and pharynx, and 3,400 deaths from cancer of the larynx. These cancers are receiving scrutiny regarding environmental factors (personal and social). Shifts in the rates in the various age and sex cohorts are being followed with interest.

Rates are interesting, but actual numbers illustrate more vividly why cancer and being old seem to go together. Table 25.3 shows the number of deaths attributed to the four leading cancer sites for males.

Table 25.3. 1977 Mortality for the four leading cancer sites for males

	All ages	75+
Lung	68,481	14,060
Colon and rectum	24,984	8,811
Prostate	20,790	11,645
Pancreas	10,938	3,205

An undue proportion of these deaths was noted in this small part of the population.

A similar notation is evident among women as shown in Table 25.4.

Table 25.4. 1977 Mortality for the four leading cancer sites for females.

	All ages	75+
Breast	34,481	8,166
Colon and rectum	26,608	11,953
Lung	22,029	4,341
Uterus	10,842	2,970

Death is a traditional end point to count from in trying to understand the phenomenon of cancer, but it omits much of the story and much of the problem, because we should all be interested in the living part of life. Frequency of deaths fails to highlight the attention on living caused by cancers ranging from the common and easily cured superficial skin cancers (approximately 300,000/yr.) to the current all-consuming therapeutic programs associated with control efforts around bone, blood, and lymphatic tumors.

Dealing with Cancer

The patient's reality is expressed as moving between four value-laden, hard-to-define words, life, death, health and disease which vary in meaning depending on age, experiences,

philosophy, culture, family, sensitivity, capacity to
function, and a host of other factors.

Unfortunately in our tradition a basic avoidance, denial
of, and technical capacity to delay death (the last enemy)
has led to some medical behavior that strays a bit away from
an idealized and holistic concept of the medical process.
Medicine can help patients in coping with certain problems.

This ideal is badly trampled in the way things actually
happen in our modern medical culture. One of my patients
drew a picture showing a group of cave men on the attack
labeled "So you have cancer, let me introduce you to my
oncologic assistants." The three leading cave men bearing
clubs are shown as surgery, radiation, and chemotherapy,
with an added note stating that the ones in the background
are yet to be fully identified. The picture is signed
with my patient's six-digit hospital number. He identifies
himself this way as he wants to highlight the impersonaliza-
tion that modern medicine with its technical requirements
for data gathering and recording requires.

The violent metaphors associated with cancer and death
have affected medical judgment and strategies. The fight
against cancer has led to many victories over cancer with
destruction of meaningful life in the person who has the
cancer.

The first step in dealing with cancer is to find and
name it. A person who is cognizant of the signals his body
sends him regarding change in function, change in weight,
bleeding, a lump, cough, or change in appearance, and who
consults with his physician has a better chance of early
detection, intervention, and perhaps management of a cancer
problem. Unfortunately, these warning signals often appear
late in the course of any cancer in terms of possibility
of cure or even containment. The name "cancer," however,
has to be applied.

All too often fatalism, pride, denial of problems, or
lack of access to a sympathetic source of medical care
pushes medical intervention into the role of dealing with
a clinical illness.

In this setting, dealing with the elderly patient with
cancer becomes complicated. The cancer itself or the many
possible associated problems in an aging patient make it
important that good medical judgment be applied and that
the patient and his family be included as much as possible
in the decisions surrounding the diagnostic and therapeutic
process. Unfortunately, clinical behavior around cancer
has often addressed the cancer problem with an insensitivity
to the patient. A study strategy called "staging" surrounds
many cancers. This is where the physician attempts to
define the cancer, first as to type then as to spread. This
process is of verying extent and is itself a burden to the
patient. Each new technology that helps us define anatomy,

physiology, or pathology tends to be used, often in an
automatic fashion irrespective of either cost or discomfort.
Although many of the new technologies are "noninvasive,"
such as studies by the Echo machine, radio nucleides, or
computerized axial tomography, some of my cancer patients
have related to me that lying still for those studies can
easily match the discomfort of barium enemas, or even bone
marrow examinations. Even more invasive staging maneuvers
such as mediastinoscopy, colonoscopy, or gastroscopy,
lymphangiography or liver biopsy often precede the major
"fight" against cancer.

As the litany of procedures, studies, and attacks
continues, you should be thinking about costs. Room, board,
and nursing care in our hospital is $100/day. Most of the
studies I listed above go for around $200 each with the CAT
scans around $300. Of course, putting the name on the cancer
requires a bit (or a lot) of the cancer itself for the surgeon to remove ($100 - $2500), the pathologist to read
($100 - $200), the radiotherapist to treat ($3,000/course)
or the oncologist to drug ($3,000/yr. for a course of drugs
plus clinic visits plus lab work).

Why do all of this? Why do any of this? Should part
of this not be done? In dealing with patients with cancer,
particularly older patients with cancer, working physicians,
who are usually younger, often lose sight of the major goals
of medicine: to care, to prevent and relieve suffering,
to do no harm, and, finally, if possible, to help restore
to health. The power that modern biologic technology has
given us (at sometimes a terrible cost) has distorted some
of these traditional goals. This has been aided and abetted
by the traditional ways we look at the problem scientifically.
If, for instance, we define success in cancer treatment as
"five-year survivals" and failure as "death," it is easy
to understand how medical values and behavior can be
distorted toward "keeping alive," with success measured in
quantity not quality of life. This distortion is made even
easier as the true costs, both monetary and life costs, are
hidden by societal values and programs.

In caring for an elderly patient with cancer, these
costs should be clearly recognized. The idea of tempering
curative attempts with simply caring and simple palliation
would perhaps help restructure society's values. As Sir
MacFarlan Burnet points out, "the insanely mounting costs
of medical care [in the past decade] . . . [have] not
significantly increased the average expectation of life
of people in their sixties and seventies" (2).

The on-line physician is still dealing with the
biological costs of cancer, which includes, among other
symptoms, to be relieved of pain, dysfunction, or bleeding.
What is he to do?

Physicians can interact with patients and their illness so that less costly and more efficacious clinical strategies toward rendering quality life can follow.

Within the framework of caring for patients with cancer, young or old, comes the reality of dealing with those approaching death. Often in older patients, this period of "predeath" is unfortunately a long, drawn out process, draining them and their loved ones of much that the preceding years of living had given. In older days travelers on a journey could find shelter and help in a hospice. The Hospice movement brought here from England is spreading across the country, with the idea that by planned, careful, professional support and organization, the terminal patient and his family can be sustained through this period, be kept free from pain, and enjoy quality life and sharing with those he loves (3). This movement is characterized by care, simplicity, emphasis on home, family and freedom from pain with reduction of medical intervention to as low a level as possible. Death from cancer under such circumstances is no longer an offence to others' sensibilities. It comes after one has time to say goodbye and is not marked by degrading pain.

Summary

Cancer is a very common problem in the elderly and a widely recognized cause of morbidity, mortality, and medical care costs. Current approaches to cancer care conceptually ignore traditional goals of medical care, such as the primacy of the relief of suffering. Redefinition and reevaluation of the real costs of good cancer care, as well as a more open understanding of the dying process, is being facilitated by better patient insight and public movements exemplified by the hospice.

References

(1) Silverberg, E. "Cancer Statistics, 1980." Ca-A Cancer Journal for Clinicians 30(1):23-38, Jan./Feb. 1980.
(2) Burnet, Macfarlan. "A Time to Die." Sciences 18:20-24, 1978.
(3) Krant, Melvin J. "The Hospice Movement." New Eng. J. of Med. 299:546-549 (Sept.) 1978.

CHAPTER 26

RENAL CHANGES WITH AGE

Ralph Goldman

The kidney increases in size during maturation, reaches a
maximum in early maturity, and then decreases in size.
The precise decrease is subject to dispute, but it appears
to be about 20%-30%. Each kidney has approximately one
million nephrons at birth and this number does not
subsequently increase, despite the fact that in some
mammals, such as the rat, there is the development of a
significant number of new nephrons prior to maturity.
After maturity there is a slow but significant nephron
loss that appears to accelerate after the sixth decade.
Ultimate loss of 30% of nephrons is an accepted figure,
although there is considerable variability. Since once
lost, either from disease or as a normal aging phenomenon,
the nephron is never replaced, it is difficult to determine
which of these two factors has caused the loss.
     Despite many obsolescent nephrons, cortical scarring
is not prominent, although it does increase with age of the
individual. Abnormal infiltrates have not been reported in
senescent kidneys in the absence of pathological processes.
Although atherosclerosis may be present in the larger blood
vessels, there is no significant evidence of focal infarctions as a cause of nephron loss. Most authors are agreed,
in the absence of hypertension, that there is no significant
change in wall:lumen   ratios and luminal diameters of small
arteries and arterioles. Small arteries and arterioles are
likely to show angulation, tortuosity, luminal irregularities
and notching at the bifurcations. Changes in the arcuate
arteries show stronger correlation with age. Capillary
basement membrane thickening has been noted by several
authors, both in the glomeruli and in the tubules.
     The most interesting interesting anatomical changes
are associated with loss of glomeruli. Details have been
defined by many investigators, but best illustrated in the
studies of Ljungqvist (1) and Takazakura (2) and their
associates. These changes are summarized in figures 26.1
and 26.2.

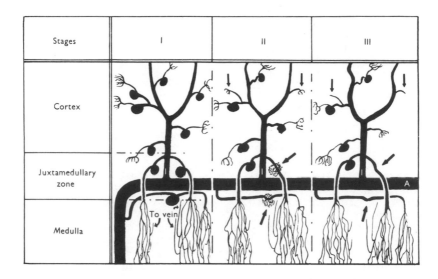

I. Interlobular artery   A. Arcuate artery

Figure 26.1

Diagram showing changes in the intrarenal arterial pattern
with age. (A. arcuate artery. I, interlobular artery.)
Stage I. Basic adult pattern showing glomerular arterioles.
Stage II. Partial degeneration of some glomeruli. Two
cortical afferent arterioles ramify into remnants of glomerular
tufts (small arrows). Two juxtamedullary arterioles pass
through partially degenerated glomeruli (large arrows). There
is slight spiraling of interlobular arteries and afferent
arterioles. Stage III. Two cortical afferent arterioles end
blindly (small arrows), and two juxtametulary tufts have
degenerated completely. The spiraling of interlobular
arteries and afferent arterioles is now more pronounced.
(From Ljungqvist, A. and C. Lagergren. "Normal Intrarenal
Arterial Pattern in Adult and Ageing Kidney. A Micro-
Angiographical and Histological Study." J. Anat. Lond.
96:285-298, 1961, by permission of the publisher, Cambridge
University Press.)

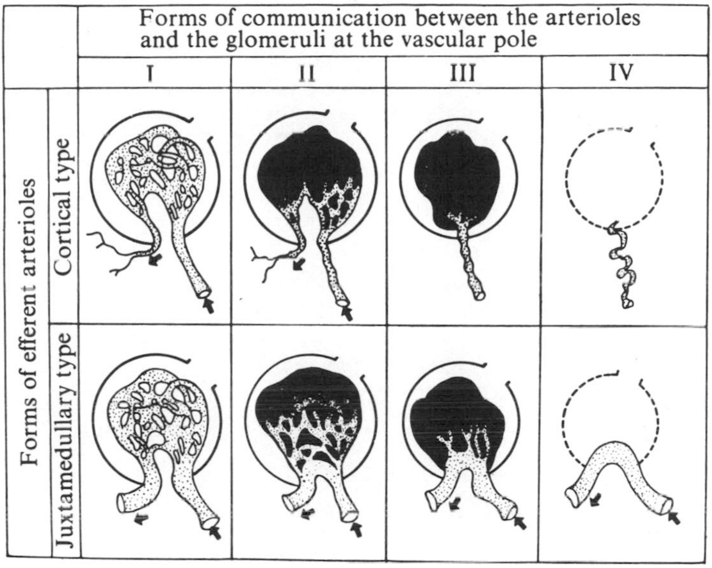

Figure 26.2

Diagram of the degeneration process in the cortical and juxtamedullary nephrons. (Reprinted from Kidney International 2:225, 1972 by permission of the publisher.)

Cortical nephrons and juxtamedullary nephrons appear to be lost by somewhat different mechanisms. The process in cortical nephrons starts in the capillary network with development of sclerotic material which obliterates the capillaries Progressive hyalinization of glomerulus takes place, but afferent arteriole remains patent and injectible for some time after loss of renal corpuscle. Eventually, hyalinized material may be reabsorbed and there may be no apparent residue of the former glomerulus. Pelvic and juxtamedullary glomeruli regress in a somewhat different manner. Hyalin material that is deposited in glomerulus is arranged so that one capillary remains as a shunt between the afferent and efferent arteriole. This capillary gradually takes on arteriolar configuration as the remainder of the glomerulus disappears. The end result is a small kink in an arteriole that goes directly from the interlobular artery to supply the tubules as the arterioli recti of Ludwig, where they then break up into a capillary plexus. According to Takazakura this shunting is seen in 9% of the juxtamedullary glomeruli at birth and increases, reaching 100% during the ninth decade. This loss of glomeruli appears to start with glomerular capillaries rather than with larger vessels, which should be the case if the process were initiated by the usual forms of atherosclerosis.

As a result of anatomic changes with age, there are
definite changes in renal function. The most thoroughly
studied change has been the decrease in glomerular filtration rate. Wesson (3) has summarized the results of many
studies of inulin clearance as shown in Figure 26.3.

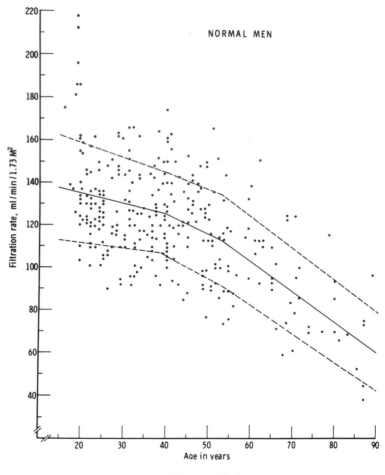

Figure 26.3

The relationship of age to the filtration rate (inulin
clearance) per 1.73m² surface area in normal men. The
solid line is the mean, by age, and the dashed lines
represent the limits of one standard deviation. (From
Wesson, Physiology of the Human Kidney, New York: Grune
and Stratton, 1969, by permission of the publisher.)

While the average decrease is approximately 0.6% per year, there is obviously an accelerating decline as age advances. A recent study reported by Rowe and his associates (4,5) indicates there is a segment of the population in whom there is no decrease in renal function for periods as long as ten years or more, raising again the question whether these decreases are a function of age or are the result of pathological processes.

In the evaluation of renal function with age, there is no significant change in level of serum creatinine (4). This results because there is a proportionate decrease in muscle mass with age and thus production of creatinine requiring excretion. Therefore, serum creatinine cannot be used as a measure of renal functional decline with age without a calculation of creatinine clearance.

There has been interest in the relationship of aging decline of glomerular filtration and dosage of drugs that are excreted primarily by filtration. A 50% reduction in filtration rate can produce significant alterations in drug requirements. However, a 50% reduction is relatively insignificant for a generation of physicians trained to manage patients with much greater degrees of renal functional impairment. Although a significant number of older individuals continue to have normal renal function, this underlines the fact that functional levels cannot be taken for granted on the basis of age alone. Therefore, as with all patients, it is necessary to individualize and to identify the level of renal function if this function is a significant factor in drug excretion.

Renal blood flow also decreases with age. Validity of the determinations of renal blood flow has been established by demonstrating that extraction ratio of para-aminohippurate is identical in the young and the old (6). However, a number of studies have indicated that the filtration fraction rises with age, indicating that renal blood flow decreases at a faster rate than does the filtration rate (7). This is a critical issue, since it can be the result of either physiologic mechanisms or of anatomic changes. Now, there are excellent studies that support both mechanisms and the problem cannot be considered resolved (8,9).

Tubular maxima for excretion of diodrast, para-amino hippurate and glucose all show declines that parallel the decline in glomerular filtration rate rather than decline in renal plasma flow. The maximum renal concentrating ability decreases with age from a maximum of 1,109 mOsm/liter in young subjects to 882 mOsm/liter in older subjects with a mean age of 68 years. The maximum specific gravity in youth of 1.030 or more decreases to a maximum of 1,023 at age 90. Although free water clearance decreases with age, and therefore minimal urinary osmolarity and specific gravity rise, free water clearance has also been found to

parallel decrease in glomerular filtration rate (10).
Finally, production of ammonia, while decreased in age,
is also found to parallel the decrease in glomerular
rate (11).

Under basal conditions, there is no change in plasma
levels of major electrolytes or of hydrogen-ion concentration.   However, because of impaired function, there is
prolongation of decrease in blood pH and bicarbonate
concentrations following an acid load.   There is also an
increase in proportion of acid load excreted as titratable
acid in comparison to that excreted as ammonium ion.

In summary, renal function of the normally aged kidney
is competent to perform its normal functions.   However,
functional reserve is impaired and must be compensated under
conditions of stress.   Since this impairment is much less
than effectively managed in many diseases with renal functional impairment, management of these problems should
present no particular difficulties if they are properly
recognized.

An interesting and perhaps significant phenomenon of
the aging kidney is the reduced capacity for compensatory
hypertrophy.   First recognized by Addis and his associates,
this now has become important because of use of donor
kidneys for renal transplantation (12, 13).   In young
individuals removal of one kidney results in sufficient
compensatory hypertrophy so final volume and function return
to 75%-80% of the original.   This response is inversely
proportionate to age, and final size and function are only
60%-65% in older individuals.   Enlargement and increase
in function is achieved by enlargement of individual
nephrons.   There is evidence that new nephrons are formed
or that there is a deceleration in the rate of loss of
existing nephrons.   Several studies indicate that nephron
enlargement is primarily at the glomerulus and proximal
convoluted tubule and that, while in younger individuals
it is associated with a cellular hyperplasia, there is
cellular hypertrophy in older individuals (14).

Most of the changes that have been enumerated are
universal and part of the general pattern of aging, not
only in the kidney but in the organism as a whole.   There
are many who believe that these changes are due to residue
of specific disease and environmental processes and are
not necessarily intrinsically derived.   This is a fascinating
and fundamental problem and it is hoped that it will be
resolved by further study (15-17).

(1)   Ljungqvist, A., and C. Lagergren. "Normal Intrarenal
      Arterial Pattern in Adult and Ageing Human Kidney. A
      Micro-Angiographical and Histological Study." J. Anat.
      Lond. 96:285-298, 1962.
(2)   Takazakura, E., N. Sawabu, A. Handa, A. Takada, A.
      Shinoda, and J. Takeuchi. "Intrarenal Vascular Changes
      with Age and Disease." Kidney International 2:224-230,
      1972.
(3)   Wesson, L. G., Jr., "Renal Hemodynamics in Physiological
      States." In Physiology of the Human Kidney, edited by
      L. G. Wesson, Jr. New York: Grune and Stratton, 1969,
      pp. 98-100.
(4)   Rowe, J. W., R. Andres, J. D. Tobin, A. H. Norris, and
      N. W. Shock. "The Effect of Age on Creatinine Clearance
      in Men: A Cross-Sectional and Longitudinal Study."
      J. Geront. 31:155-163, 1976.
(5)   Shock, N. W., R. Andres, A. H. Norris, and J. Tobin.
      Patterns of Longitudinal Changes in Renal Function."
      Abstracts for 11th International Congress of Gerontology,
      August 20-25, 1978, Tokyo, Japan, p. 142.
(6)   Miller, J. H., R. K. McDonald, and N. W. Shock. "The
      Renal Extraction of P-Aminohippurate in the Aged
      Individual." J. Geront. 6:213-216, 1951.
(7)   Davies D. F., and N. W. Shock. "Age Changes in
      Glomerular Filtration Rate, Effective Renal Plasma
      Flow, and Tubular Excretory Capacity in Adult Males."
      J. Clin. Invest. 29:496-507, 1950.
(8)   McDonald, R. K., D. H. Soloman, and N. W. Shock.
      "Aging as a Factor in the Renal Hemodynamic Changes
      Induced by a Standardized Pyrogen." J. Clin. Invest.
      5:457 462, 1951.
(9)   Hollenberg, N. K., D. F. Adams, H. S. Solomon, A.
      Rashid, H. L. Abrams, and J. P. Merrill. "Senescence
      and the Renal Vasculature in Normal Man." Circulation
      Res. 34:309-316, 1975.
(10) Lindeman, R. D., T. D. Lee, Jr., M. J. Yiengst, and
      N. W. Shock. "Influence of Age, Renal Disease, Hyper-
      tension, Diuretics, and Calcium on the Antidiuretic
      Responses to Suboptimal Infusions of Basopressin."
      J. Lab. Clin. Med. 68:206-223, 1966.
(11) Adler, S., R. D. Lindeman, M. J. Yiengst, E. Beard,
      and N. W. Shock. "Effect of Acute Acid Loading on
      Urinary Acid Excretion by the Aging Human Kidney."
      J. Lab. Clin. Med. 72:278-289, 1968.
(12) MacKay, L. L., E. M. MacKay, and T. Addis. "Influence
      of Age on Degree of Renal Hypertrophy Produced by High
      Protein Diets." Proc. Soc. Exp. Biol. 24:335, 1926.

(13) Boner. G., W. D. Shelp, M. Newton, and R. E. Rieselbach.
      "Factors Influencing the Increase in Glomerular
      Filtration Rate in the Remaining Kidney of Transplant
      Donors." Am. J. Med. 55:169-174, 1973.
(14) Mandache, E., and E. Repciuc. "Microautoradiographic
      Study of Cell Proliferation in Compensatory Renal
      Growth." Morphol. Embryol. Physio. 21:71-78, 1975.
(15) Goldman, R. "Aging of the Excretory Systems: Kidney
      and Bladder." In Handbook of the Biology of Aging,
      edited by C. E. Finch and L. Hayflick. New York:
      Van Nostrand Reinhold, 1977, pp. 409-431.
(16) Lindeman, R. D. "Age Changes in Renal Function."
      In The Physiology and Pathology of Human Aging, edited
      by R. Goldman and M. Rockstein. New York: Academic
      Press 1975, pp. 19-38.
(17) McLachlan, M. S. F. "The Aging Kidney." Lancet
      2:143-145, 1978.

CHAPTER 27

URINARY TRACT INFECTIONS AMONG THE ELDERLY

Charles J. Schleupner

Urinary tract infections comprise a spectrum of clinical
entities whose common denominator is the presence of bacteriuria. These infections occur throughout life, primarily
in females, but reach their peak prevalence among the
elderly (1, 2). This change in prevalence is a reflection
of complex and multiple interactions occurring during the
aging process. This paper will include a brief review of
the epidemiology, pathogenesis and etiology of cystitis
and pyelonephritis in the elderly, along with comments
about their diagnosis and management. The topic of
prostatitis will also be briefly discussed, but a review
of urethritis will not be attempted.

EPIDEMIOLOGY

The prevalence of bacteriuria among adult females rises from
1%-4% before age 50 to 10%-15% after the sixth decade of
life. Among adult males, the low incidence of bacteriuria
before age 50 (less than 1%) has been shown in some surveys
to rise in the 60- to 70-year age group to levels comparable
to the female population. After age 60 the incidence of
symptomatic infection among males may actually exceed that
of females (1). Despite these data, Williamson et al.,
have shown that family physicians are unaware of the presence
of chronic urinary tract infections in many of their
patients (3). A reemphasis of the frequent occurrence of
urinary infections among the aged is needed.
    Along with the aging process, debility plays a signifi-
cant role in the acquisition of urinary infections (4).

Table 27.1. Incidence of urinary infection in the elderly in relation
             to residence.

Residence	Incidence (%)		Age group (Years)
	Men	Women	
Living at home	3	12	60-65
Living at home	10	23	$\geq$65
Nursing home residents	26	23	>70
Acute care hospital admissions	33	32	>70
Long-term care patients	34	34	>65

Source: Adapted from Lye, M. *Geriatrics* 33:71-77, 1978.

As shown in Table 27.1, while the incidence of urinary
tract infections increases with age among the elderly who
reside at home, this incidence increases at an even greater
rate for similarly aged men and women who are nursing home
residents or patients in acute care or long-term-care
hospital settings. Others have confirmed these data (5, 10).

PATHOGENESIS AND PATHOPHYSIOLOGY

While prolonged immobilization associated with debility may
result on bone demineralization, hypercalciuria, and stone
formation, these sequelae account for only a small number
of urinary infections related to debility. Other more
significant factors predisposing the elderly to urinary
tract infections are outlined as follows.

1. Diminished reponse to stress
2. Poor nutritional status
3. Decreased cell-mediated immunity
4. Decline of IgG and IgM levels
5. Chronic diseases
    a. Diabetes mellitus
    b. Chronic renal disease
    c. Malignancies
    d. Use of cytotoxic agents, steroids and
       radiation therapy
6. Chronic prostatitis
7. Diminished outflow from the urinary bladder
   due to
    a. Urethral stenosis, cystoceles
    b. Prostatic hypertrophy
    c. Prostatic carcinoma
    d. Bladder diverticuli or tumors
    e. Neurogenic bladder
8. Urinary calculi
9. Vesicoureteral reflux
10. Indwelling urinary catheters
11. Other genitourinary instrumentation.

The elderly have a diminished response to stress and
have a higher incidence of poor nutrition, which may relate
to the damped or delayed cell mediated immune responses in
vitro and in vivo observed among the elderly (7, 8).
Polymorphonuclear leukocyte functions, which may more
directly relate to urinary tract defenses, have been found
to be intermittently abnormal in the aged who do not have
malignant disease (8) and more consistently abnormal in
those with myeloproliferative and lymphoproliferative
disorders (15). A decline of circulating IgG and IgM levels
in the aged has been found by some investigators (8, 15).
These findings may relate to the increased incidence of
urinary tract infections, at least among elderly females;
Stamey et al. have related the absence of cervicovaginal

antibody (IgA, IgG and IgM) against endogenous fecal flora
to recurrent bacteriuria in females (9).

A number of chronic disease states, in part due to
accompanying debility, have been associated with an increased
incidence of urinary tract infections (6). Specifically,
patients with diabetes mellitus appear to have a higher
incidence of pyelonephritis, while their overall rate of
urinary tract infections does not differ from a control
population. Factors causally related to their increased
incidence of pyelonephritis are abnormalities of polymorphonuclear leukocyte function associated with hyperglycemia
and frequency of urinary catheterization in this group of
patients. The increased incidence of renal infection in
patients with chronic renal disease cannot be explained by
their increased frequency of instrumentation and is probably
related to deficient local defense mechanisms within the
kidney itself (6). Associations of increased frequency of
urinary tract infections with malignancies and the use of
chemotherapeutic agents are probably indirectly due to
related complications and their management.

In males recurring urinary tract infections are frequently related to chronic bacterial prostatitis, which presents a difficult therapeutic problem because antimicrobials
penetrate the prostate poorly, thereby allowing survival of
bacteria which subsequently reinfect the urine (2, 6, 34).
Although acute bacterial prostatitis may precede chronic
bacterial prostatitis, most men are unaware of a previous
acute episode (34). While some patients are asymptomatic,
most complain of varying amounts of dysuria, urgency, frequency, nocturia, low back and perineal discomfort, myalgias
and/or arthralgias (34). Occasional accompanying low grade
fever is more frequent with acute exacerbations of chronic
prostatitis. In addition to recurrent cystitis, upper
urinary infections and epididymitis are also complications
of chronic bacterial prostatitis. Regardless of the presence
of chronic bacterial prostatis, the loss of the antibacterial
activity of prostatitic secretions with aging has also been
invoked to explain the increased incidence of urinary
infections in elderly males (4).

Anatomical factors and abnormal bladder physiology
often relate to the occurrence of urinary infections.
Throughout life females are predisposed to the acquisition
of urinary infections due to their shorter urethral length
and the lack of prostatic secretions which have antibacterial activity (2, 4, 6). Additionally, obstruction to
urinary outflow and incomplete emptying of bladder are
frequent and important causes of urinary tract infections
in the elderly. These abnormalities may be related to
urethral stenosis (due to prior instrumentation or surgery),
the presence of cystoceles, prostatic hypertrophy or
carcinoma, urinary bladder diverticuli or tumors, or central

nervous system disease with secondary bladder dysfunction
(2, 6, 31). Abnormal cystometrograms have been documented
in elderly women with and without central nervous system
disorders (31). Incomplete emptying of urinary bladder
may result from any of these abnormalities and thereby
impair mechanical washout, which is the bladder's most
effective defense mechanism against infection. Secondary
urinary stasis allows for replication of microorganisms
and local infection. Additionally, some authors believe
that bladder distention results in bladder wall ischemia
and a secondary reduction of local resistance to infection
with consequent tissue invasion (4, 13). The presence of
urinary or prostatic calculi, frequently composed of
magnesium ammonium phosphate or calcium phosphate, harbors
bacteria that are difficult to eradicate and present
therapeutic problems because of the high frequency of
recurrent infection. Furthermore, the presence of urinary
calculi may result in urinary obstruction and lead to sepsis
and destruction of renal parenchyma (6). While vesicoureteral reflux is common in children as a result of
urinary infection, its occurrence in the adult often
signifies the presence of a congenital abnormality or
severe bladder distention (2, 6). Whatever the cause,
reflux allows for bacteria from the lower urinary tract
to enter the upper tract with resultant renal infection.
        Urinary catheterization and other genitourinary
instrumentation and surgery, often necessary procedures in
the elderly, allow for ready entry of microorganisms and
account for many hospital-acquired urinary infections
(2, 6, 10). Even a single brief urethral catheterization
for diagnostic purposes in hospitalized or bedridden patients
carries a greater risk of subsequent bacteriuria (5%-10%)
than the same procedure in healthy outpatients, which is
associated with only a 1%-3% risk (1, 6). With meticulous
attention to maintainance of a closed urinary drainage
system during continuous urinary catheterization, the risk
of bacteriuria is 50% at 10 days, but eventually all patients
will develop bacteriuria with continued catherization (6,
11). Furthermore, recent evidence shows that antibiotic
irrigation of the catheter and bladder may not reduce this
rate of acquisition of infection (12).

ETIOLOGIC AGENTS

With this background about the factors predisposing the
elderly to urinary tract infections, a comparison of the
etiologic agents of urinary tract infections in the young
and aged adult population is presented in Table 27.2.

Table 27.2. Frequency of organisms isolated from different population
            groups with urinary tract infections

Organism	Young men	Frequency (%) in each population		
		Elderly in community	Elderly in Hospital	
			Men	Women
E. Coli	75	78	29	52
Proteus	8	7	50	20
Klebsiella	4	2	0	1
Pseudomonas	1	2	4	2
Staphylococcus	6	3	5	2
Others	6	8	12	10

Source: Adapted from Lye, M. Geriatrics 33:71-77, 1978.

      An individual's own enteric flora are believed to
colonize the perineal and periurethral areas and result in
urinary infections. The presence of fecal incontinence
among the elderly due to dementia and other forms of central
nervous system dysfunction may further predispose this group
to urinary infections. The role of introital colonization
by fecal flora in the pathogenosis of recurrent urinary
infections in females has been demonstrated by Stamey et
al. (9). These findings are corroborated by the fact that
E. coli causes 75%-80% of urinary infections in young adults
and ambulatory elderly patients (2, 4, 6). However, other
Gram-negative organisms, including Proteus spp., Pseudomonas
aeruginosa, and members of the Klebsiella-Enterobacter
family, assume importance among the elderly who are hospitalized. The reason for the predeliction of Proteus spp.
for elderly males is unclear. This organism is also
associated with an alkaline urine and urinary calculus
formation due to its urea-splitting property. Undoubtedly,
involvement of resistant Gram-negative isolates in hospital-
acquired and recurrent urinary infections is a reflection
of antimicrobial induced selection. While enterococci
also play a role in urinary infections among the elderly,
Candida spp., Trichomonas vaginalis, Chlamydia trachomatis,
Ureaplasma urealyticum and viruses (adenovirus, mumps virus,
cytomegalovirus and measles virus) are not usual pathogens
in this age group.

CLINICAL MAINFESTATIONS

Symptoms occasionally associated with acute cystitis in the
elderly are: (1) painful (burning) micturition; (2) urgency,
frequency; (3) lower abdominal pain; (4) incontinence;
(5) occasionally, confusion in the elderly.

While dysuria, urgency, frequency, lower abdominal
pain, and incontinence have classically been linked with
lower urinary tract infection, Brocklehurst et al. found no
symptoms which correlated with the presence of urinary
infection among 172 elderly males (10). Furthermore, only
precipitancy and difficulty in urination were linked with
lower urinary infection among 334 elderly females in their
study; noteworthy was a lack of correlation of frequency,
incontinence, or nocturia with urinary infection for either
sex. Interestingly, confusion in an elderly individual may
occasionally be the sole manifestation of lower urinary
infection (4). The absence of specific symptoms in this
age group undoubtedly accounts for the lack of physician
awareness of urinary infections among the elderly (3). An
appropriate caveat in geriatric medicine is "to consider
urinary infection whenever an unexplained change in clinical
status occurs."

Symptoms and signs of pyelonephritis are as follows.
1.   Acute Pyelonephritis
     a.   Dysuria, frequency
     b.   Rigors, fever and toxicity
     c.   Flank pain; may be absent in the elderly
     d.   Bacteremia and shock
2.   Chronic Pyelonephritis
     a.   Low-grade fever, malaise, weight loss, or
     b.   Same symptom complex as with acute pyelonephritis
     c.   Often without classic symptoms and may be
          asymptomatic.

While acute pyelonephritis appears to be uncommon in
the elderly (4), the same cautions about anticipating a
typical complex of signs and symptoms for cystitis in the
elderly applies as well for acute pyelonephritis. Dysuria
and frequency are unreliable indicators of any urinary
infection in the aged; however, even rigors, fever, systemic
toxicity, and flank pain, while often present, may be mild
or absent in elderly individuals with acute pyelonephritis
due to their poor response to stress. The physician's
attention may first be gained by the patient's manifestations of dehydration (4, 6). Elderly patients may be
bacteremic and lapse into septic shock with minimal signs
or symptoms. Furthermore, the symptoms and signs of acute
pyelonephritis may abate after several days despite continued infection. The latter observation is believed to be
a manifestation of patient tolerance to endotoxin, believed
to be the mediator of many of the classical signs and

symptoms of this syndrome (6). Therefore, both appropriate
diagnosis and documentation of adequacy of therapy require
bacteriologic support.

Chronic pyelonephritis in the elderly is often insid-
ious, though it may present with the same symptom complex
typical of acute pyelonephritis. More often, patients
either complain of malaise, weight loss, low grade fever,
recurrent urinary tract infections, or have symptoms of
urinary obstruction. Moreover, they may be entirely asymptomatic and the disease discovered due to an abnormal
urinalysis or an elevated blood urea nitrogen. Chronic
pyelonephritis should be suspected in any patient who has
chronic bacteriuria associated with obstruction to urine
flow or a neurogenic bladder.

DIAGNOSIS

Approach to diagnosis of urinary tract infections in
the elderly does not differ from that used in younger adults
and depends upon the demonstration of significant bacteriuria
by quantitative culture of an appropriately collected specimen. After discarding the first 10 ml. of voided urine, a
midstream specimen should be collected in a sterile con-
tainer. Patients require instruction about careful cleansing
of the periurethral area before voiding. More detailed discussions of these procedures can be found elsewhere (1, 16).
However, despite careful instruction, the elderly may be
less able to comply than younger adults due to declining
mental and physical abilities. Lye has noted that 57% of
midstream urine specimens obtained from elderly women are
falsely positive (4). Furthermore, Stamey et al. have shown
(Table 27.3) that, of 54 females (age unstated) with
sterile urine obtained via suprapubic bladder aspiration,
only one (1.9%) could void a sterile midstream urine specimen after careful instruction (16).

Table 27.3. Midstream urine bacterial counts in 54
females with sterile suprapubic urinary
bladder aspirates

Bacteria/ml.	Percent of total patients
Sterile	1.9
1-100	16.7
100-1,000	38.9
1,000-10,000	24.1
10,000-100,000	11.1
> 100,000	7.4

Source: Adapted from Stamey et al. Medicine 44:1-36,
1965.

Perhaps more significantly, 4 (7.4%) of these women with sterile suprapubic aspirates voided urine specimens containing greater than 10^5 organisms per ml. In contrast, when 151 females with sterile suprapubic bladder aspirations were aided by a nurse in obtaining midstream urine specimens for culture, 54 (36%) were able to void a sterile urine specimen and none voided a urine contaminated with $\geq 10^5$ organisms. It is clear that the care with which a voided urine specimen is obtained from any population of patients, especially the elderly, will have a direct influence upon the accuracy of the culture results obtained and upon the appropriateness of care rendered. All of these comments presume prompt handling of these specimens, which is another necessity for appropriate interpretation of culture results.

Table 27.4.   Methods for the diagnosis of significant bacteriuria

---

1. Clean-catch midstream urine culture with $\geq 10^5$ organisms/ml. of one species in the female
    a. One specimen: 80% specificity if asymptomatic
                         diagnostic if symptomatic
    b. Two specimens: 92% specificity if asymptomatic
    c. Three specimens: 98% specificity if asymptomatic
2. Midstream urine culture with $\geq 10^4$ organisms/ml. of one species in the male
    a. One specimen: diagnostic if symptomatic
    b. Two specimens: diagnostic if asymptomatic
3. Urine culture obtained by urethral catheterization containing $\geq 10^4$ organisms/ml. of one species
4. Urine culture obtained by suprapubic aspiration should be sterile.

As shown in Table 27.4, criteria for diagnosis of significant bacteriuria vary depending upon the sex of the patient, presence or absence of symptoms, and method of collection. For the asymptomatic female, one midstream urine culture containing $\geq 10^5$ organisms per ml. of one species is diagnostically accurate in 8 out of 10 occasions. Second and third specimens containing similar numbers of the same species of organism increase specificity, as shown in Table 27.4. At least two specimens are necessary for the diagnosis of asymptomatic bacteriuria in the female (2). If a female is symptomatic, a single midstream urine culture containing $\geq 10^5$ organisms per ml. of one species is acceptable diagnostically, but acquisition of a second specimen is ideal (12). For the asymptomatic and symptomatic male, similar criteria apply to a midstream urine culture, except most authorities will accept $\geq 10^4$ organisms per ml. as a quantitative criterion (2, 14). If a brief urethral catheterization is necessary to obtain urine for culture, the presence of >10^4 organisms per mil. of one species is diagnostic of a urinary infection (14). As mentioned, the risk of secondary bacteriuria developing related to this procedure must be considered when it is elected. In this regard, suprapubic bladder aspiration, an underutilized procedure in adult and geriatric medicine, can obviate the risks associated with a brief urethral catheterization and provide the most reliable urine specimen for diagnostic culture. Any growth in such a specimen is significant, but, in the presence of a urinary infection, organism numbers usually exceed 5,000 per ml. of urine (1, 2, 14, 16). This procedure, described elsewhere, is often less traumatic to the patient than urethral catheterization (16).

The presence of polymicrobic bacteriuria in any urine specimen should suggest inappropriate collection or handling of the specimen. Should adequately collected specimens consistently reveal multiple identical pathogens in significant numbers in the absence of a chronic urinary catheter or ileal bladder, serious urinary tract pathology should be suspected (2, 4, 6). Additionally, the quantitative criteria outlined in Table 27.4 apply to common Gram-negative bacilli only. Quantitative criteria have not been established for Gram-positive and other more fastidious bacteria or the fungi (2); these organisms commonly do not replicate to high titers, and, when cultured, their significance must be established with repeated specimen collection.

In addition to quantitative urine culture, there are numerous screening tests for bacteriuria as reviewed by Kunin, suitable for use in office practice or for performing surveys and which have varying degrees of sensitivity and specificity (17). The presence of greater than five leukocytes per high power microscopy field in the sediment of a centrifuged urine specimen has a variable correlation with the presence of urinary infection. The detection of one or more bacteria in the Gram stained smear of a drop of uncentrifuged, freshly voided urine has been shown to have an 80%-90% correlation with the presence of >10^5 organisms per ml. of urine (32, 33). Recently, the presence of one or more bacteria per oil immersion microscopy field in each of five fields examined using uncentrifuged, unstained urine or >10^4 leukocytes per ml. of uncentrifuged urine had been shown to correlate well with urinary infection (18, 19). However, these techniques are tedious and impractical for routine use.

While the presence of a urinary tract infection can be documented with appropriately obtained urine cultures, the differentiation of renal from bladder infection is often difficult on the basis of symptoms and signs alone, especially in the elderly; however, the distinction is therapeutically important. The presence of a positive blood culture containing a pathogen identical to that in the urine culture in the absence of recent lower urinary tract instrumentation defines with high probability a renal source for the infection. In addition, there are a number of indirect and direct techniques for making this distinction which have been described and reviewed elsewhere (1, 6, 13, 16). Each of these techniques is associated with significant inaccuracies or risks; perhaps the most practical and rewarding is the bladder washout technique (1). The most promising recent development is an indirect test which determines the presence or absence of antibody-coated bacteriuria (20, 21). The presence of immunoglobulin coating bacteria present in the urine correlated well with the presence of renal infection, while its absence defined lower urinary tract infection However, subsequent studies have shown lesser degrees of sensitivity and specificity (22-24). The adaptation of this technique to daily clinical use may be important in the future.

THERAPY

Preliminary comments about the therapy of urinary infections in the elderly are appropriate. The rate of adverse drug reactions is higher in elderly adults compared to their younger counterparts. This results primarily from their decreased renal excretory capacity due to both intrinsic renal disease and obstructive uropathy (2, 15). Additionally, a decreased lean body weight, often present in the elderly, may result in overdosage with potentially toxic, lipid insoluble aminoglycoside antimicrobials, which are often required to treat the more resistant Gram-negative isolates encountered in these patients. While elimination of urinary infection in the elderly is no more difficult than in comparable younger adults, the frequency of recurrence is higher. If symptomatic, this implies the possibility of repeated exposure to potentially toxic antimicrobials with each recurrence. Therefore, it is important to choose not only an antimicrobial to which the pathogen is sensitive, but also one which is least toxic and has the most narrow spectrum of activity to avoid selection of more resistant organisms (2, 6). Generally, bactericidal agents are preferred over bacteristatic drugs to reduce the need for retreatment. Duration of therapy should be minimized while being efficacious.

Acute Infections

In addition to the above considerations, the decision must be made whether to treat an individual patient. Every episode of symptomatic bacteriuria in the elderly should be treated (2, 4, 6). With regard to the first episode of

acute cystitis, oral therapy with a sulfonamide (e.g.,
sulfisoxazole), ampicillin, nitrofurantoin, or, in the case
of pencillin allergy, a cephalosporin would be reasonable
due to the likelihood of a sensitive E. coli in this setting
(2, 6, 15). Culture results may necessitate a revision of
this choice. Therapy should be continued for no more than
seven to ten days (2); some studies suggest the efficacy of
a single dose or up to a three-day course of therapy with
uncomplicated acute cystitis (2,6). An often forgotten
adjunct to antimicrobial therapy is the use of urinary
analgesics for symptomatic relief. While urine cultures
should be sterile at 48 hours after initiating therapy (2),
follow-up cultures should be obtained two weeks after discontinuing therapy and, when there is a risk of renal damage
with a recurrence, at six weeks and six months after therapy
is completed (2, 15).

Recurrent Infections

The potential outcomes of therapy for an acute symptomatic
urinary infection can be defined as: (a) cure, (b) persistence of the infecting organism throughout therapy,
(c) relapse, indicating disappearance of the infecting
organism during therapy, followed by its recurrence within
two weeks of discontinuing therapy, and (d) reinfection
with the same or another organism, usually within six
months of therapy (2). The causes of bacterial persistence
and relapse are outlined as follows: (1) organisms were
initially or have become resistant to the antimicrobial
used; (2) therapy inadequate; (3) antimicrobial chosen was
not excreted in the urine; (4) infected renal calculi;
(5) chronic bacterial prostatitis; (6) renal parenchymal
infection (pyelonephritis); (7) urinary structural abnormalities or obstructive uropathy; (8) cell wall deficient
organisms.
      Bacterial persistence or relapse usually reflects
therapy with an antimicrobial to which the organism is not
sensitive, an inadequate course of therapy, use of an agent
which is not excreted in the urine (possibly due to renal
failure), or the presence of renal calculi, prostatitis,
pyelonephritis, urinary structural abnormalities, or
obstruction (2, 6). The development of cell wall deficient
organisms during therapy accounting for recurrent infections
is largely a theoretical concern and has only been demonstrated for enterococci (25). Persistence or relapse of
infection justifies therapy, whether it is symptomatic or
asymptomatic (2, 6). In addition to alteration of previously inappropriate or inadequate therapy and performance
of appropriate urologic, radiographic, and surgical
evaluation, some authors believe that patients with persistence or relapse of a urinary infection after a brief

course of therapy should be treated for three to six weeks
with an antimicrobial to which their infecting organism is
sensitive (2, 6). In the case of a male with prostatitis,
a frequent cause of relapsing infection or apparent reinfection, up to three months of therapy with trimethoprim-
sulfamethoxazole may be indicated (26).

Reinfection after initial therapy of a urinary infection is seen more often in females and has been related to
colonization of the introital area with their endogenous
fecal flora (2, 6, 9). Infrequent, symptomatic reinfections
in women (no more frequently than two per year) should be
treated as acute episodes with a seven-day course of an
appropriate antimicrobial (2). Long-term, low-dose trimethoprim-sulfamethoxazole prophylaxis (half tablet daily
or every other day for six months) after initial specific
therapy against the infecting organism has been shown to
decrease significantly more frequent symptomatic reinfections in women (27). Efficacy in this setting is apparently
related to the ability of trimethoprim to enter vaginal
secretions and reduce introital colonization with potential
pathogens. While the appearance of drug-resistant organisms
has not been a problem, such women should be followed
monthly for a recurrence of symptoms or with urine culture
to monitor for the emergence of resistant organisms (2).

While advice concerning reinfection bacteriuria in the
female seems to have a rational basis, our understanding of
this problem in the male is less clear and the recommendations more complex. The most complete recent study of
chronic bacteriuria in males (both symptomatic and asymptomatic) and its therapy was performed by a United States
Public Health Service sponsored program that evaluated 249
men with reinfection or "late relapse" of bacteriuria (25).
This study revealed that: (a) long-term prophylactic therapy for chronic bacteriuria delays, but does not prevent,
the recurrence of bacteriuria after an initial course of
organism-specific therapy; (b) urologic sepsis was prevented
in the group receiving prophylaxis; and (c) in the absence
of severe urologic abnormalities or noninfectious renal
disease, chronic bacteriuria was unrelated to the progression of renal failure. After data analysis these authors
recognized a number of good and poor prognostic signs that
can be used as a guide to the management and therapy of
elderly males with bacteriuria (Table 27.5).

Table 27.5. Patient characteristics of value in predicting response
            to therapy in bacteriuric men

Good prognosis

Symptoms present 12 months or less
No previous therapy for UTI
Normal prostate clinically and radiologically
Normal IVP
Pure Escherichia coli infection

Poor prognosis

Definite	Possible
Calculus disease of the upper urinary tract	Symptoms for 20 years or more
Prostatic calculi	Four or more previous courses of therapy for UTI
Focal renal atrophy with sub-jacent calyceal deformity	Prostatic enlargement clinically and radiologically
Mixed infection	Recurrent bacteriuria with the same organism (relapse)
Enterococcal infection	Serum creatinine, 2 mg./100 ml. or more

---

Source: Adapted from Freeman, R. B., et al. Ann Intern Med 83:133-
         147, 1975.

They concluded that men with infrequent recurrences of
symptomatic bacteriuria should be treated briefly with
organism-specific therapy for each recurrence if they have
all of the good prognostic factors listed in Table 27.5 and
none of the poor prognostic factors. The authors additionally recommended that, regardless of symptoms, any elderly
male with infrequent recurrences of bacteriuria and "possible" poor prognostic signs should be managed with short-term,
specific therapy and careful follow-up urine cultures
without continued prophylaxis. They also concluded that
men with frequent recurrences of symptomatic bacteriuria
and males with two or more of the "possible" poor prognostic
factors or with a "definite" poor prognostic factor (Table
27.5) should be considered for continued prophylaxis after
a brief, specific course of therapy. The decision for
prophylaxis must be made after consideration of the potential
benefits and toxicities from such therapy, especially if
there is preexisting renal compromise. Alternative agents
to trimethoprim-sulfamethoxazole for prophylaxis of recurrent, symptomatic infections in both elderly men and women
include nitrofurantoin (50 to 100 mg daily), sulfisoxazole
or sulfanethoxazole (500 mg daily), and methanamine
mandelate (2 grams daily, with ascorbic acid, 2 grams daily).
     Any consideration of the therapy of recurrent urinary
tract infection in elderly males must deal with the therapy

of chronic bacterial prostatitis, which is associated
causally with these recurrences. Meares has shown that two
tablets twice daily of trimethoprim-sulfamethoxazole given
for 12 weeks permanently cured one-third of a group of 16
patients with chronic bacterial prostatitis documented by
segmented localization cultures of lower urinary tract
specimens (34). While this regimen is the most effective
current therapy, Fair et al. have recently challenged the
theoretical basis for its success and have proposed a re-
appraisal of other antimicrobials for use in this setting
(35).

Despite considerable past debate, many authorities
today agree that asymptomatic bacteriuria should not be
treated in elderly patients who do not have those poor
prognostic signs outlined in Table 27.5 (2, 4, 25). The
reasons include the lack of definitive evidence for deterioration of renal function in this subset of the elderly
despite untreated bacteriuria and the frequency of isolation
of drug-resistant organisms which require the use of
potentially toxic antimicrobials (2, 25, 28). Should the
urinary bacterial isolate in this circumstance be sensitive
to nontoxic agents, some authorities have favored therapy
for 10-14 days (15). Furthermore, there is agreement that
in any patient with chronic bacteriuria in whom urinary
tract instrumentation is planned, organism-specific antimicrobial therapy should precede the procedure with the
goal of sterilization of the urine in order to minimize the
likelihood of a secondary bacteremia.

While acute pyelonephritis is uncommon among the
elderly (4), its therapy is no different from that in other
age groups (6). Depending upon the severity of illness, an
individual without a prior history of urinary infection,
urologic abnormalities, or instrumentation may be treated
in the outpatient or inpatient setting (6). Therapy for
an initial episode of pyelonephritis without signs of
systemic toxicity can be treated on an outpatient basis
with oral sulfonamides, tetracycline, ampicillin, nitrofurantoin, or a cephalosporin given for 10-14 days (6). A
prior history of urinary problems dictates the need for
hospitalization because of the possibility of the presence
of an antimicrobial-resistant organism, which necessitates
that initial therapy be parenteral with broad-spectrum
agents (usually ampicillin or a cephalosporin plus an
aminoglycoside). Patients who relapse after initial oral
or parenteral therapy should be retreated for six weeks with
an antimicrobial to which the organism remains sensitive,
while appropriate urologic and radiologic evaluations are
completed (6).

The management of chronic pyelonephritis necessitates
complete urologic and radiologic evaluation of the urinary
tract (6). Organism-specific therapy frequently requires

a parenteral antimicrobial because selection of resistant organisms by frequent prior treatments has occurred. If the urine culture is sterilized within 72 hours of initiation of therapy, specific antimicrobials should be continued for 10 days, when the patient should be placed on an oral agent for a minimum of 3 months (e.g., trimethoprimsulfamethoxazole, nitrofurantoin, or methanamine mandelate with ascorbic acid). Periodic urine cultures should be obtained during continuous therapy. Results of therapy for chronic pyelonephritis may be gratifying because of the reversal and improvement of deteriorating renal function seen with successful treatment.

Catheter-associated Infections

Comments about the management of catheter-associated bacteriuria are especially relevant in the discussion of urinary infections in the elderly due to their frequent debility requiring prolonged catheterization. The rate of acquisition of bacteriuria during indwelling urethral catheterization was defined previously (11). Guidelines for catheter placement and maintenance are thoroughly discussed elsewhere (1, 29). Once a patient has acquired bacteriuria despite adherence to these guidelines, as is inevitable with increased duration of catheterization (11), only acute symptomatic infections should be treated with organism-specific antimicrobials (6). Therapy of asymptomatic, monomicrobic bacteriuria with bacterial suppressants (methenamine mandelate, nitrofurantoin, or a sulfanomide) may be elected (20), but such therapy may be readily justified for catheter-associated polymicrobic bacteriuria because of its recently documented association with spontaneous bacteremia (30). Additionally, any manipulation of a urinary catheter in the presence of bacteriuria should be preceded by organism-specific therapy.

From the foregoing information, the complexities related to the pathophysiology and management of urinary tract infections in the elderly are evident. The subtle symptom array suggesting the diagnosis of these infections emphasizes the need for a high index of suspicion when caring for the aged and may partially account for the unusually high prevalence (79%) of undocumented urinary infections in the survey of Williamson et al. (3). The diagnosis and management of urinary infections, annoying and often overlooked afflictions in the elderly, offer an example of the challenge and potential gratification to the internist practicing geriatric medicine.

References

(1)   Kunin, C. M. Detection, Prevention and Management of
      Urinary Tract Infections. 2d ed. Philadelphia: Lea
      & Febiger, 1974.
(2)   Santoro, J., and D. Kay. "Recurrent Urinary Tract
      Infections: Pathogenesis and Management." Med. Clin.
      N. Amer. 62:1005-1020, 1978.
(3)   Williamson, J., I. H. Stokoe, S. Gray, M. Fisher,
      A. Smith, A. McGhee, and E. Stephenson. "Old People at
      Home: Their Unreported Needs." Lancet 1:1117-1120,
      1964.
(4)   Lye, M. "Defining and Treating Urinary Infections."
      Geriatrics 33:71-77, 1978.
(5)   Klarskov, P. "Bacteriuris in Elderly Women." Dan.
      Med. Bull. 23:200-204, 1973.
(6)   Riff, L. J. M. "Evaluation and Treatment of Urinary
      Infections." Med. Clin. N. Amer. 62:1183-1199, 1978.
(7)   Palmer, D. L. and W. P. Reed. "Delayed Hypersensitivity
      Skin Testing, II: Clinical Correlates and Allergy."
      J. Infect. Dis. 130:138-143, 1974.
(8)   Phair, J. P., C. A. Kauffman, A. Bjornson, J. Gallagher,
      L. Adams, and E. V. Hess. "Host Defenses in the Aged:
      Evaluation of Components of the Inflammatory and Immune
      Responses." J. Infect. Dis. 138:67-73, 1978.
(9)   Stamey, T. A., N. Wehner, G. Mihara, and M. Condy.
      "The Immunologic Basis of Recurrent Bacteriuria: Role
      of Cervicovaginal Antibody in Enterobacterial Coloni-
      zation of Introital Mucosa." Medicine 57:47-56, 1978.
(10) Brocklehurst, J. C., J. B. Dillane, L. Griffiths, and
      J. Fry. "The Prevalence and Symptomatology of Urinary
      Infection in an Aged Population." Geront. Clinica
      10:242-253, 1968.
(11) Garibaldi, R. A., J. P. Burke, M. L. Dickman, and
      C. B. Smith. "Factors Predisposing to Bacteriuria
      during Indwelling Urethral Catheterization." New
      Eng. J. Med. 291:215-219, 1974.
(12) Warren, J. W., R. Platt, R. J. Thomas, B. Rosner, and
      E. H. Kass. "Antibiotic Irrigation and Catheter-
      associated Urinary Tract Infections." New Eng. J. Med.
      299:570-573, 1978.
(13) Merritt, J. L. "Urinary Tract Infection, Causes and
      Management, with Particular Reference to the Patient
      with Spinal Cord Injury: A Review." Arch. Phys.
      Med. Rehab. 57:365-373, 1976.
(14) Meares, E. M., Jr. "Asymptomatic Bacteriuris: Current
      Concepts in Management." Postgrad. Med. 62:106-111,
      1977.
(15) Gladstone, J. L. and R. Recco. "Host Factors and
      Infectious Diseases in the Elderly." Med. Clin. N.
      Amer. 60:1225-1240, 1976.

(16) Stamey, T. A., D. E. Govan, and J. M. Palmer. "The
      Localization and Treatment of Urinary Tract Infections:
      The Role of Bactericidal Urine Levels as Opposed to
      Serum Levels." Medicine 44:1-36, 1965.
(17) Kunin, C. M. "New Methods in Detecting Urinary Tract
      Infections." Urol. Clin. N. Amer. 2:423-432. 1975.
(18) Barbin, G. K., J. D. Thorley, and J. A. Reinarz.
      "Simplified Microscopy for Rapid Detection of Signifi-
      cant Bacteriuria in Random Urine Specimens." J.
      Clin. Microbiol. 7:286-291, 1978.
(19) Musher, D. M., S. B. Thorsteinsson, and V. M. Airola,
      II. "Quantitative Urinalysis: Diagnosing Urinary
      Tract Infection in Men." J.A.M.A. 236:2069-2072, 1976.
(20) Thomas, V., A. Shelokov, and M. Forland. "Antibody-
      Coated Bacteria in the Urine and the Site of Urinary-
      Tract Infection." New Eng. J. Med. 290:588-590, 1974.
(21) Jones, S. R., J. W. Smith, and J. P. Sanford.
      "Localization of Urinary-Tract Infections by Detection
      of Antibody-Coated Bacteria in Urine Sediment." New
      Eng. J. Med. 290:591-593, 1974.
(22) Rumans, L. W., and K. L. Vosti. "The Relationship of
      Antibody-Coated Bacteria to Clinical Syndromes as
      Found in Unselected Populations with Bacteriuria."
      Arch. Intern. Med. 138:1077-1081, 1978.
(23) Harding, G. K. M., T. J. Marrie, A. R. Ronald, S.
      Hoban, and P. Muir. "Urinary Tract Infection Localiz-
      ation in Women." J.A.M.A. 240:1147-1150, 1978.
(24) Hawthorne, J. J., S. B. Kurtz, J. P. Anhalt, and J. W.
      Segura. "Accuracy of Antibody-Coated-Bacteria Test
      in Recurrent Urinary Tract Infections." Mayo Clin.
      Proc. 53:651-654, 1978.
(25) Freeman, R. B., W. M. Smith, J. A. Richardson, P. J.
      Hennelley, R. H. Thurm, C. Urner, J. A. Vaillancourt,
      R. J. Griep, and L. Bromer. "Long-Term Therapy for
      Chronic Bacteriuria in Men: U.S. Public Health Ser-
      vice Cooperative Study." Ann. Intern. Med. 83:133 117,
      1975.
(26) Meares, E. M. "Long-Term Therapy of Chronic Bacterial
      Prostatitis with Trimethoprim-Sulfamethoxazole." Can.
      Med. Assoc. J. 112:22S-25S, 1975.
(27) Stamey, T. A., M. Condy, and G. Mihara. "Prophylactic
      Efficacy of Nitrofurantoin Macrocrystals and Trimetho-
      prim-Sulfamethoxazole in Urinary Infections: Biologic
      Effects on the Vaginal and Rectal Flora." New Eng.
      J. Med. 296:780-783, 1977.
(28) Gleckman, R. "The Controversy of Treatment of
      Asymptomatic Bacteriuria in Non-Pregnant Women--
      Resolved." J. Urol. 116:776-777, 1976.
(29) Stamm, W. E. "Guidelines for Prevention of Catheter-
      Associated Urinary Tract Infections." Ann. Intern.
      Med. 82:386-390, 1975.

(30) Gross, P. A., M. Flower, and G. Barden. "Polymicrobic
      Bacteriuria: Significant Association with Bacteremia."
      J. Clin. Microbiol. 3:246-250, 1976.
(31) Brocklehurst, J. D., and J. B. Dillane. "Studies of
      the Female Bladder in Old Age, II: Cystometrograms in
      100 Incontinent Women." Geront. Clinica 8:306-319,
      1966.
(32) Bulger, R. J., and W. M. Kirby. "Simple Tests for
      Significant Bacteriuria." Arch. Intern. Med. 112:
      742-746, 1963.
(33) Kass, E. H. "Asymptomatic Infections of the Urinary
      Tract." Trans. Assoc. Am. Physicians 69:56-63, 1956.
(34) Meares, E. M., Jr. "Prostatitis: A Review." Urol.
      Clin. N. Amer. 2:3-27, 1975.
(35) Fair, W. R., D. B. Crane, N. Schiller, and W. D. W.
      Heston. "A Re-Appraisal of Treatment in Chronic
      Bacterial Prostatitis." J. Urol. 121:437-441, 1979.

CHAPTER 28

TREATMENT OF END-STAGE RENAL DISEASE IN THE AGED

Jorge Roman

In treatment of end-stage renal disease (ESRD), three basic modalities (1) are available and are used either alone or in various combinations:

1. Conservative management includes general medical measures, such as diets, prescription of activity level, drugs, and management of complications and intercurrent illnesses.

2. Dialysis, including both hemo and peritoneal dialysis, can offer life support even in stages of renal failure where conservative measures alone are insufficient.

3. Renal transplantation, when successful, can reinstitute all normal kidney functions and thus provide the best quality of life for ESRD patient.

Historically, conservative measures have been used since Richard Bright's time. With understanding of need to restrict protein intake in the 1920s and 1930s and later with Rose's (2), Giordano's (3), and Giovanetti's (4) work on diets emphasizing proteins of high biological value, dietetic management developed into the current era. Better understanding of metabolism and definition of requirements for different salts, vitamins, and calories have allowed a more rational basis for dietetic prescriptions in renal failure (5). Dietetic requirements, however, have not been well defined for the aging population with ESRD and may prove different from younger subjects.

There is still some controversy over the role of severely limited diets in practical management of ESRD, since while they can control symptoms and may delay need for replacement therapy, often they are poorly tolerated and can lead to malnutrition that delays recovery once dialysis is started (6).

With widespread availability of dialysis in this country, many clinicians now prefer to use minimally restricted diets and start dialysis earlier. In the early years of chronic dialysis, it was a rule not to offer chronic dialysis unless the creatinine clearance was less than 3 ml/min and creatinine (serum) above 15. Now it is not uncommon to start dialysis with clearances between 5 and 10 ml/min and serum creatinine around 10. It is argued that such patients will be less symptomatic and fare better on dialysis, but comparative studies are lacking.

Another important milestone in conservative management was better understanding of calcium/phosphorus/vitamin D metabolism (7). Currently, use of binders to lower serum phosphorus is started much earlier in renal failure than a few years ago.

Conservative measures are used on all patients regardless of age. Since they are part of standard medical practice and relatively inexpensive, most aged renal failure patients have access to them.

A few special problems in dietetic management in aged should be noted. Protein-restricted diets are unappealing and require major changes in eating habits. If special foods are prescribed, costs are very high and tastes and textures can be unfamiliar and unappealing, thus diminishing compliance. In our program, a full-time dietician works with each patient, not only to prescribe a diet, but to monitor actual compliance and check intake records.

The main problems we have encountered in the aged is anorexia and insufficient intake, as opposed to younger patients where diet excess is the main problem. In order to assure sufficient nutrition and to prevent tissue wastage, many times we liberalize the diet, by allowing either extra foods or even full "free," i, e., uncontrolled, meals on a periodic basis, to assure overall compliance and nutrition. Alcohol can be allowed in moderate quantities, if not abused. It may improve appetite and food tolerance.

Phosphorus binders (Al(OH)3, aluminum carbonate, are of help in controlling secondary hyperparathyroidism (8). They uniformly induce severe constipation; therefore, a stool softener (Diocytol, Calcium Sulfosuccinate, Sorbitol) must be used preventively.

The best conservative measures can only prolong life if some kidney function remains, but in progressive renal disease, sooner or later, support therapy is needed. Dialysis and transplantation are those therapies.

Although one of Kolff's first patients was a lady with ESRD, chronic dialysis was not attempted for ESRD until 1962 (9), when development of arteriovenous shunts allowed long-term vascular access. Chronic peritoneal dialysis (10) was not possible until more permanent access devices were designed, first by Palmer and Quinton (11) and later by Tenckhoff (12).

Since dialysis was very effective in prolonging life, and even allowing a rather high quality of independent life, but very expensive (13), resources proved totally inadequate to meet the demand. High costs and the limited number of centers forced strict patient selection. For this purpose "selection committees" were organized in all centers and selection criteria drafted (14-15).

Age was the first criterion considered, limiting patients to under age 50 or even age 45. Other excluding criteria employed were medical, such as history of hypertension, myocardial infarction, diabetes mellitus, and cerebrovascular disease. Others were social criteria such as potential for rehabilitation, self-care, social worth, and others.

In the past fifteen years two developments have dramatically changed chronic dialysis from a research tool
available to a few selected patients to a commonly practiced
therapy. First, dialysis itself has changed, by developing
better vascular access devices (AV fistulas) (16), by
developing better hardware and disposables, and by learning
better how to use them. With these, in spite of accepting
older and more infirm patients, mortality has been reduced
to about 15% in the first years and 8% thereafter (17), but
just as important, quality of life for the dialysis patient
has dramatically improved.

In parallel, funding has become available in most indus-
trialized countries allowing expansion of programs to meet
increasing demand. Currently, dialysis is a common procedure that cannot be denied to any patient because of age,
funding, or lack of resources, and patients and families
are demanding it.

Another important development is peritoneal dialysis,
which can replace, sometimes advantageously, hemodialysis
and can be done at home during sleep or even continuously
(18), during normal waking hours without any equipment.

The number of patients eligible for dialysis has
increased rapidly, reflecting both a lowering of "selection
criteria," especially age, and uncovering a large reservoir
of patients that formerly died, their deaths ascribed to
other causes. Today up to 130 patients per million population per year are judged potential candidates for chronic
dialysis (19).

Early reports emphasized high mortality of the aged in
center hemodialysis. For example, Pendras et al. (Seattle (20)
reported in 1970 60% mortality in those over age 56 as
opposed to 15% in those under that age at two years into
dialysis. In contrast, in 1978 reported mortalities by
Lebkiri et al. (Hospital Necker) (21) at two years are
9.5% for patients under age 50 and 20.6% in those above Bovy
et al.(22) in Liege reported the same, meeting no significant
mortality difference in patients above age 50, followed to
three years into chronic center hemodialysis. In the more
aged population, patients over age 70, Chester et al. (23)
(Georgetown) reported at two years 58% mortality as opposed
to 42% in patients under age 42, with less survival of
those dialysis patients who remained hypertensive on
dialysis.

The trend to improved survival on chronic dialysis is
best reflected in two longitudinal studies. Sreepada-Rao
et al. (24) in patients over age 50 reports a decrease in
annual mortality from 46% in 1973 to 13.5% in 1977, with
a marked increase in percentage of new patients over age
50, from 28% in 1973 to 68% in the past two years.

Walker et al. (25) with same age cut-offs, reports 92%
survival in the first year and 64% at three years, compared

with 70% survival for patients under age 50. Survival drops
to 30% vs 68% at five years. In this group a striking
difference is observed in survival of aged patients in
receiving in-center hemodialysis versus those on home hemodialysis, with survival at three years of 48% vs 28% for
in-center. This could reflect patient selection or effects
of treatment.

In our program we do not find any significant differences, on most patients under age 55, but in a few over age
60 (about 15% of total) vascular access and problems with
volume changes during dialysis are encountered. Vascular
sclerosis can be associated with decreased fistula survival
and peripheral "steal syndrome" can occur.

Rapid volume changes during rapid hemodialysis can lead
to hypertension, with arrythmias, myocardial infarctions,
and transient ischemia attacks, or, on the other hand, pulmonary edema. Careful volume replacement can control these
complications in most patients. Since we use glucose-free
dialyzate, hypoglycemia can occasionally occur.

Home training for patients above age 55 has been difficult in our experience, with slow training in hemodialysis
techniques, but this is linked both to patient and partner
limitations.

In contrast, peritoneal dialysis appears to be a better
treatment for the aged. Vascular access is not needed,
except to provide an alternative to treatment. Peritoneal
catheters (Tenckhoff type) are easily placed at bedside and
maintained. Training is easier and fewer skills required
before home dialysis can be started, leading to shorter
training times and a lower failure rate.

The main problem with peritoneal dialysis continues to
be peritonitis (26), with about one episode per patient, per
year, and eventual failure of peridialysis, leading to
hemodialysis. Since peritoneal dialysis is very slow,
blood pressure tends to remain constant or change very
slowly during the procedure. Dialyzate contains glucose,
so hyperglycemia rather than hypoglycemia can occur. The
gradualness of changes in peridialysis allows asymptomatic
treatments, so well tolerated that they are usually done at
night, unattended.

Development of continuous ambulatory peritoneal
dialysis (CAPD) (27) is foreseen as ideal for aged patients,
since constant blood chemistries and ease of procedure allow
greatest patient well being. It is not yet in widespread
application, but some workers foresee one-third of all
patients receiving CAPD (28).

There is yet scant data as to the results of long-term
chronic peridialysis in aged. One of the few large groups
was reported by Fenton et al. (29) from Toronto General. They
electively place patients over age 60 on peridialysis,
mainly at home. Of their total patient population, this age

group constitutes 33% of the peridialysis patients, while only 7.5% of the hemodialysis group are over age 60. In their initial report they note a higher mortality in peridialysis, 31% per patient/year, as compared with 14% per patient/year on hemodialysis. This finding is unique and has not been explained.

Transplanting kidneys into aged recipients is also very new. Related living grafts are few since siblings are also likely to be old, and grafts from children to parents are not used in many centers.

A report from Portland, Oregon (30), concludes that allografting with cadaveric kidneys has a survival equal to dialysis, but their definition includes as higher age group ages 45 to 57 years. Within that age, cumulative survival up to five years was similar for both groups, while quality of life was much better for the grafted group. As of now, there are no reports of risks of transplanting patients over age 60, but most groups discourage this procedure (31).

Currently used immunodepressive therapies have many side effects, including increasing risk and severity of infections, development of Cushing's Syndrome, and bone damage. They may be more severe in elderly.

In the United States special problems develop concerning transportation to and from dialysis centers.

It is difficult to foresee future developments in such a new field, but possibilities include widespread usage of CAPD, allowing ambulatory treatment of many patients without machines or disruption to life-style. Oral treatments, including sorbents by mouth, such as resins to bind potassium, oxycellulose, and others may allow reducing frequency of dialysis. (32). Hybrid treatment regimens, combining more aggressive diet management, sorbants by mouth with various peri- and hemo-dialysis, may also allow simpler and safer dialysis. Even sweating regimens may find a role in future patient management (33).

In the future, less toxic immunodepressive regimes, combined with greater availability of kidneys, may allow cadaveric allografting to be used more, even in the aged patient.

198   Health Care of the Aging

References

(1)   Friedman, Eli A., ed. Strategy in Renal Failure.
      New York: John Wiley & Sons, 1978.
(2)   Rose, W. C. "The Aminoacid Requirements of Adult Man."
      Nutr. Abstr. Rev. 27:631, 1957.
(3)   Giordano, C. "Use of Exogenous and Endogenous Urea for
      Protein Synthesis in Normal and Uremic Subjects."
      J. Lab. & Clin. Med. 62:231-246,
      1963.
(4)   Giovannetti, S., and Q. Maggiore. "Low Nitrogen Diet
      with Proteins of High Biological Value for Severe
      Chronic Uremia." Lancet 1:1000-1003, May 9, 1964.
(5)   Berlyne, G. M. "Dietary Treatment of Chronic Renal
      Failure." In Strategy in Renal Failure, edited by
      E. A. Friedman. New York: John Wiley & Sons, 1978,
      pp. 175-185.
(6)   Manis, T. "Maintenance Hemodialysis." In Strategy
      in Renal Failure, edited by E. A. Friedman. New York:
      John Wiley & Sons, 1978, pp. 209-235.
(7)   Avioli, L. V., and S. L. Teitelbaum. "The Renal
      Osteodystrophies." In The Kidney, edited by Barry M.
      Bremmer and F. L. C. Rector. Philadelphia: W. B.
      Saunders, 1976, pp. 1542-1591.
(8)   Bricker, N. S. "On the Pathogenesis of the Uremic
      State: An Exposition of the 'Trade-Off Hypothesis.'"
      New Engl. J. Med 286:1093-1099, 1972.
(9)   Quinton, W. E., D. H. Dillard, J. J. Cole, and B. H.
      Scribner. "Eight Months' Experience with Silastic-
      Teflon Bypass Cannulas." Trans. Am. Soc. Artif. Intern.
      Organs 8:236-245, 1962.
(10) Rae, A., and M. Pendray. "Advantages of Peritoneal
      Dialysis in Chronic Renal Failure." J.A.M.A. 225:937-
      941, 1973.
(11) Palmer, R. A., W. E. Quinton, and J. E. Gray. "Pro-
      longed Peritoneal Dialysis for Chronic Renal Failure."
      Lancet 1:700-702, March 28, 1964.
(12) Tenckhoff, H., and H. Schecter. "A Bacteriologically
      Safe Peritoneal Access Device." Trans. Am. Soc. Artif.
      Intern. Organs 14:181-187, 1968.
(13) Oberley, E. T., and T. D. Oberley. "Adjustment and
      Rehabilitation." In Understanding Your New Life with
      Dialysis, Springfield, Ill.: Charles C. Thomas
      Publishers, 1975.
(14) Alexander, S. "They Decide Who Lives, Who Dies."
      Life 53: 102-104, Nov. 9, 1962.
(15) Fox, R. S., and J. P. Swazey. The Courage to Fail, 2d
      ed., rev. Chicago: University of Chicago Press 1978,
      pp. 226-344.

(16) Brescia, M. J., J. E. Cimino, K. Appel, and B. J.
      Hurwich. "Chronic Hemodialysis Using Venipuncture
      and a Surgically Created Arteriovenous Fistula,"
      N. Engl. J. Med. 275:1089-1092, 1966.
(17) Roberts, S. D., D. R. Maxwell, and T. L. Gross. "Cost
      Effective Care of End Stage Renal Disease: A Million
      Dollar Question." Ann. Intern. Med. 92:243-
      248, 1980.
(18) "The Body May Be Best." Time 112:82, December 18,
      1978.
(19) Burton, B. T. "Overview of End Stage Renal Disease."
      J. Dial. 1:1-23, 1976-77.
(20) Pendras, J. P., and T. L. Pollard. "Eight Years
      Experience with a Community Dialysis Center: The
      Northwest Kidney Center." Trans. Am. Soc. Artif.
      Intern. Organs 16:77-84, 1970.
(21) Lebkiri, B., L. Boudier, A. Lemaire, N. K. Man, and
      P. Jungers. "Hemodialyse Periodique chez le sujet
      age: Experience Favorable chez 22 Patients Ages de
      plus de 60 ans." VIIth Int. Congress Neph. Abstracts,
      S-25, Montreal, Canada, 1978.
(22) Bovy, P., C. Remy, and G. Porive. "Chronic Hemodialy-
      sis in Elderlies." VIIth Int. Congress Neph. Abstracts,
      S-24 Montreal, Canada, 1978.
(23) Chester, A., A. Giacalone, T. Rakowski, W. P. Argy,
      and C. E. Schreiner. "Hemodialysis in the 8th and 9th
      Decade of Life." VIIth Int. Congress Neph. Abstracts,
      S-20, Montreal, Canada, 1978.
(24) Sreepada-Rao, T. K., S. R. Hirsch, and E. A. Friedman.
      "Striking Increase in Older and Diabetic Patients on
      Maintenance Hemodialysis in Brooklyn." VIIth Int.
      Congress Neph. Abstracts, V-3, Montreal, Canada, 1978.
(25) Walker, P. J., H. E. Ginn, H. K. Johnson, W. J. Stone,
      P. E. Teschan, D. Latos, D. Stouder, E. L. Lamberth,
      and K. O'Brien. "Long Term Hemodialysis for Patients
      over 50." Geriatrics 31:55-61, (September) 1976.
(26) Oreopoulos, D. G. Editorial, "The Coming of Age of
      Continuous Ambulatory Peritoneal Dialysis." Dialysis
      and Transplantation 8:#5: 460, 461, 512, 1979.
(27) Popovich, R. P., J. W. Moncrief, K. D. Nolph, A. J.
      Ghods, Z. J. Twardowski, and W. K. Pyle. "Continuous
      Ambulatory Peritoneal Dialysis." Ann. Intern. Med.
      88:449-456, 1978.
(28) Oreopoulos. Editorial, "The Coming of Age," p. 460.
(29) Fenton, S. S. A., D. C. Cattran, N. Barnes, and B.
      Lewis. "Home Peritoneal Dialysis versus Hemodialy-
      sis." VIIth Int. Cong. Neph. Abstracts, S-26,
      Montreal, Canada, 1978.
(30) Golper, T. A., J. M. Barry, W. M. Bennett, and G. A.
      Porter. "Primary Cadaver Kidney Transplantation in
      Older Patients: Survival Equal to Dialysis." Trans.
      Am. Soc. Artif. Intern Organs 24:282-287, 1978.

(31) ESRD Network 30, Transplant Committee Report.
      Richmond, Va. May, 1979.
(32) Friedman, E. A. "Future Treatments of Renal Failure."
      In Strategy in Renal Failure. New York: John Wiley
      and Sons, 1978, pp. 521-548.
(33) Lacher, J. W., and R. W. Schrier. "Sweating Treatment
      for Chronic Renal Failure." Nephron 21:255-259, 1978.

CHAPTER 29

PRESCRIBING FOR THE GERIATRIC PATIENT

Richard W. Lindsay

This paper will discuss prescribing for the geriatric
patient. As the number of elderly patients increase, the
importance of prescribing also increases. By the year
2000 approximately 20%-25% of our population will be over
age 65. About 10% are now over age 65 and they receive 25%
of all out-of-hospital medications.

Prescribing for institutionalized geriatric patients
has also assumed importance, since the number of nursing
home beds is now greater than the number of acute hospital
beds.

Seidl and his associates studied a group of hospitalized elderly patients and found adverse drug reaction
in 24% of those patients over age 80, compared with 12%
in ages 40-50 (1).

Caranasos et al. observed that 3% of University of Florida
Hospital admissions were direclty related to drug-induced
illness. Over 40% of his patients were over age 60.
Drugs most frequently involved in these admissions were
aspirin, Warfarin, Digoxin, and Hydrochlorothiazide, all
commonly prescribed medications (2)

A predisposing factor for the increased rate of
adverse drug reactions among elderly patients is the high
incidence of multiple chronic diseases. Some nursing home
patients have been shown to have eight or more major disease
processes. Therefore, it is not difficult to understand
the potential and need for multiple drug utilization.
Cluff et al. (1964) have suggested a relationship between
the number of drugs taken and the percentage of adverse
reactions. In their studies, if a patient was receiving
one to five medications, he had approximately a 3%-4% chance
of an adverse drug reaction. If the individual received
eleven to fifteen medications, the rate of adverse reactions climbed to approximately 30% (3). In some nursing
home situations, medication lists approximate these figures.

Recent research questions how aging alters body
physiology and how this altered physiology affects the
actions of drugs. Perhaps studies concerning absorption,
distribution, and excretion of drugs in geriatric patients
will answer these questions. Most of the results relating
to absorption reported to date have shown conflicting
results in terms of the effect of aging on the rate of
absorption of certain drugs and chemicals. Other workers
studying the problems of drug distribution pointed out the
importance of changes in body composition on drug levels.
As an example, plasma albumin may be reduced in the older

subject. Since many medications are bound to albumin in
the plasma, decreased albumin in the older patient will
result in a greater amount of free drug and a greater
therapeutic or toxic effect. In the area of drug binding,
there is a problem caused by drug competition for binding
sites. For instance, Phenylbutazone has been shown to
displace Dilantin from its binding site and thereby increase
the amount of free Dilantin. There is a greater potential
in geriatric patients for altered drug responses, since
they frequently are receiving multiple medications and hence
have an increased chance for interactions.

     Regarding alterations in drug-excretion rates that
occur with aging, there are more reliable data available.
In a given patient the level of creatinine clearance may
vary considerably, but it is known that in some patients
the drop in creatinine clearance between ages 20 and 90 may
approximate 50%. Therefore, it is easy to understand how
higher blood levels of renally excreted drugs could result.
Elderly patients sometimes receive additional drugs whose
toxicity may further decrease renal function. An example
of such toxic drugs would be the aminoglycoside group of
antibiotics.

     One of the major factors involved in the altered rates
of drug absorption, distribution, and elimination in the
geriatric population is an alteration in tissue sensitivity.
Tissue sensitivity may change under a number of circumstances, such as malnutrition, presence of chronic disease,
etc.

     Depression is being diagnosed more frequently in the
elderly. Treatment of depression is resulting in a syndrome
that is secondary to the anticholinergic properties of the
major drugs involved in treating depression in this age
group. The tricyclic antidepressants, which include
Amitryptaline, Thioradiazine, and Desipramine, are most
frequently involved. The latter drug is reported to have
weaker anticholinergic effects than the two previous ones
and hence may be a better choice in the elderly. The syndrome itself can be seen in perhaps 5% of patients who
receive tricyclic antidepressants. Its severity may vary
from specific anticholinergic effects, such as dry mouth
or sweating, to more severe symptoms in the elderly, such
as glaucoma, cardiac manifestations including arrythmias,
postural hypotension, and urinary retention. However, where
large doses of tricyclics have been ingested, a vast array
of neuropsychiatric signs and symptoms may mimic depression
or signs of depression for which the patient is being
treated. These signs could include anxiety, agitation,
restlessness, purposeless movements, overactivity, delirium,
disorientation, and impairment of immediate and recent
memory. Obviously, major clues will be found in the patient's physical exam and here one would detect tachycardia

and arrhythmia, large sluggish pupils, flushed warm dry skin, increased temperature, decreased mucosal secretion, urinary retention, and reduced bowel motility. Therefore, we must be aware of the potential problem with toxic manifestations in utilizing these drugs and realize that it may be difficult to evaluate the patient's response because of possible toxicity.

In conclusion, here are some ways to prevent some problems of toxicity. First, one should follow the old rule of Primum non nocere, "First, do no harm." In treating elderly patients, you should be slow to add new medications, and this should only be done when the indications are present. You should attempt to maintain these patients on the lowest possible dose and be continually on the lookout for signs of toxicity. In addition, the sensitive physician will also be attuned to the fact that in many older patients socioeconomic factors may be responsible for noncompliance with medications. Therefore, when one is looking for a desired effect, one must be certain that the patient is in fact receiving the prescribed medication before adding additional dosage increments. We should also be extremely meticulous in taking a drug history in the elderly patient. In all instances, questions relating to the use of over-the-counter preparations, either in the home or, in some instances, when the patient is hospitalized, must be asked. Many of these over-the-counter preparations do, in fact, contain anticholinergic ingredients, two examples of which are sleep medications and cold remedies. Both of these could magnify the anticholinergic syndrome.

Spend additional time counseling the spouse or other responsible family members regarding the therapeutic regimen you are planning for the elderly patient. The physician should also provide this responsible individual with a copy of the proposed regimen. I use a drug calendar approach on which I list the days of the month, days of the week and actually affix specific tablets to the calendar for color comparison purposes. I also like to add specific notations as to the purpose of each tablet, such as "heart pill," "fluid pill," etc. It is also valuable to keep with each patient's chart an up-to-date drug list, notations of when the prescription was written, the number of tablets prescribed, and the number of refills required. This is of invaluable help, particularly when discussing problems with family or patients over the telephone. Simplify the drug regimens whenever possible.

Have periodic drug destruction days, during which patients and their families are asked to bring in all medications currently being utilized. On these days many medications can be found that are outdated and some that were prescribed for totally unrelated problems. Appropriate educational counseling of the family and patient regarding hazards of outdated medications is important. One of the most important roles a physician can play in geriatric prescribing is to assess continually the indications and needs for specific medications, much as we have done for the institution of new medications. This is appropriate in the chronic care setting, such as nursing homes, where drug discontinuation rounds assume major importance.

The pharmacist can be of assistance in the area of compliance both with instructions to the patient and his family and also by clear labeling of the drug containers. Stress to the pharmacist that he use large type to print the label and also that he not place the medication in a type of vial which precludes access by elderly patients with disorders such as arthritis.

The physician should utilize dietary means of meeting certain geriatric needs, such as electrolyte replacement. Milk is a good source of high potassium, as is orange juice, etc. This may assist somewhat in overcoming the patient's low fixed income and his drug costs.

References

(1)   Seidl, L. G., G. F. Thornton, J. W. Smith, and L. E. Cluff. "Studies on the Epidemiology of Adverse Drug Reaction, III: Reactions in Patients on a General Medical Service." Bull. of Johns Hopkins Hosp. 119:299-315, 1966.
(2)   Caranasos, G. J., R. B. Stewart, and L. E. Cluff. "Drug-Induced Illness Leading to Hospitalization." J.A.M.A. 228:713-717, 1974.
(3)   Cluff, L. E., C. F. Thornton, and L. G. Seidl. "Studies on the Epidemiology of Adverse Drug Reactions, I: Methods of Surveillance." J.A.M.A. 188:976-983, 1964.

Bibliography

Drug Utilization and Adverse Reactions in the Elderly

Bender, A. D. "Effect of Age on Intestinal Absorption: Implications for Drug Absorption in the Elderly." J. Am. Geriatr. Soc. 6:1331-1339, 1968.

Caranasos, G. J., R. B. Stewart, and L. E. Cluff. "Drug-induced Illness Leading to Hospitalization." J.A.M.A. 228:713-717, 1974.

Cluff, L. E., C. F. Thornton, and L. G. Seidl. "Studies on the Epidemiology of Adverse Drug Reactions, I: Methods of Surveillance." J.A.M.A. 188:976-983, 1964.

Davison, W. "Drug Hazards in the Elderly." Clin. Pharm. 6:83-95, 1971.

Freeman, J. T. "Some Principles of Medication in Geriatrics." J. Am. Geriatr. Soc. 22:289-295, 1974.

Lamy, P. P., and M. E. Kitler. "Drugs and the Geriatric Patient." J. Am. Geriatr. Soc. 19:23-33, 1971.

Lamy, P. P., and R. E. Vestal. "Drug Prescribing for the Elderly." Hosp. Practices 11:111-118 (January) 1976.

Schwartz, D. "The Elderly Patient and His Medications: Chance and Mischance." Geriatr. 20:517-520, 1967.

Seidl, L. G., G. F. Thornton, J. W. Smith, and L. E. Cluff. "Studies on the Epidemiology of Adverse Drug Reaction, III: Reactions in Patients on a General Medical Service." Bull. Johns Hopkins 119:299-315, 1966.

Smith, J. W., L. G. Seidl, and L. E. Cluff. "Studies on the Epidemiology of Adverse Drug Reaction, V: Clinical Factors Influencing Susceptibility." Ann. Intern. Med. 65:629-640, 1966.

Triggs, E. J., and R. L. Nation. "Pharmacokinetics in the Aged: A Review." J. Pharmacokinetics & Biopharmaceutics 3:387-418, 1975.

Physiologic Changes of Aging and Their Effects on Prescribing

American Pharmaceutical Association. Evaluations of Drug Reactions, 2d ed. Washington D.C.: American Pharmaceutical Association, 1976.

Anderson, W. F. Practical Management of the Elderly. Oxford: Blackwell Scientific Publications, 1971.

Bender, A. D. "The Effects of Increasing Age on the Distribution of Peripheral Blood Flow in Man." J. Am. Geriatr. Soc. 13:192-198, 1965.

Bender, A. D. "Pharmacologic Aspects of Aging: Additional Literature." J. Am. Geriatr. Soc. 15:68-74, 1967.

Bender, A. D. "Pharmacodynamic Principles of Drug Therapy in the Aged." J. Am. Geriatr. Soc. 22:296-303, 1974.

Ewy, G. A., G. G. Kapadia, L. Yao, M. Lullin, and F. I. Marcus. "Digoxin Metabolism in the Elderly." Cir. 39:449-453, 1969.

Goldman, R., and M. Rockstein (eds). The Physiology and
    Pathology of Human Aging. New York: Academic Press,
    1975.
Gorrod, J. W. "Absorption, Metabolism and Excretion of
    Drugs in Geriatric Subjects." Geront. Clinica
    16:30-42, 1974.
Vestal, R. E., E. A. McGuire, J. D. Tobin, R. Andres, A. H.
    Norris, and E. Mezey. "Aging and Ethanol Metabolism."
    Clin. Pharm. & Therap. 21:343-354, 1977.
Vestal, R. E., A. H. Norris, J. H. Tobin, B. H. Cohen, N. W.
    Shock, and R. Andres. "Antipyrine Metabolism in Man:
    Influence of Age, Alcohol, Caffeine, and Smoking."
    Clin. Pharm. & Therap. 18:425-432, 1975.

Compliance and Prevention in Geriatrics Prescribing

Anderson, W. F. "Administration, Labelling and General
    Principles of Drug Prescription in the Elderly."
    Geront. Clinica 16:4-9, 1974.
Arthur, M. B. "Formulation of Drugs for the Elderly."
    Geron. Clinica 16:25-29, 1974.
Forbes, J. A. "Prescribing for the Elderly in General
    Practice and the Problems of Record Keeping."
    Geront. Clinica 16:14-17, 1974.
Gibson, I. I. J. M. "Hospital Drugs in the Home."
    Geront. Clinica 16:10-13, 1974.
MacLennan, W. J. "Drug Interactions." Geront. Clinica
    16:18-24, 1974.
Schwartz, D., M. Wang, L. Zwitz, and M. E. Goss. "Medi-
    cation Errors Made by Elderly, Chronically Ill
    Patients." 52:2018-2029, 1962.
Stewart, R. B., and L. E. Cluff. Commentary, "A Review of
    Medication Errors and Compliance in Ambulant Patients."
    Clin. Pharm. & Therap. 13:463-468, 1972.
Wandless, I., and J. W. Davie. "Can Drug Compliance in the
    Elderly Be Improved?" Brit. Med. J. I:359-361,
    February 5, 1977.

CHAPTER 30

THE CLINICAL APPROACH TO THE GERIATRIC PATIENT

Eugene A. Stead, Jr.

During my entire professional career, a number of the
elderly have been my patients. Having been responsible
for my mother and father during their declining years and
now having medical responsibility for a kindly, confused
mother-in-law in her 91st year of life, I was content with
my knowledge of the medical needs of the aged. Three and
a half years ago I became medical director and doctor to
the Methodist Retirement Home located on the edge of the
Duke campus. Two hundred and twenty-five retired elderly
persons live in rooms, in apartments, and in this facility
for care of the aged. There are 125 nursing beds mostly
filled from the Durham Home and Lumberton, North Carolina,
Methodist Home.

On my assuming these responsibilities, an open meeting
with members of the home was held. I told them I had never
cared for old folk en masse and had a lot to learn, but if
they had a little patience they could teach me what I needed
to know. Most of them quizzed me over the years as to how
they were doing and whether I was learning. I replied they
were good instructors and I was an apt pupil. The home was
in good order! Caring for 350 old people en masse taught me
things one doesn't learn when he cares for old people
scattered throughout a practice.

This was rewarding group. They were church-going,
Godly people blessed with good manners. On a casual visit
one would never suspect the degree of confusion that existed.
Everyone cared for somebody and each one said, "Good morning.
How are you? It's a nice day." We had few smokers and no
drug or alcohol problems.

These people had reached the point where they needed
some help in their daily activities. Apartment dwellers
mostly cared for themselves, but they needed assistance not
available from their families or their community when they
became ill. The degree of loss of independence increased
as one moved to the main building and, eventually, to the
section designated as home for the aged. Dependence
increased again in the intermediate nursing unit and reached
its greatest degree in the skilled care unit.

My job was to be certain that this progressive loss of
independence could not be stayed by medical science and was
not increased by fears of professionals that people might
hurt themselves or by fears of the family for safety of
their kin. Mine was the role of friend and doctor to residents in the home. Families were met and the functional
state of new residents was reviewed with them, as well as
the role of the doctor and nurses in the home.

These people had had good medical care before they
entered the home. Few medical diagnoses were made on
admission that led to improvement in their performance.
We found some instances of hypothyroidism and Parkinsonism,
which responded to appropriate therapy. We gradually
decreased all drugs that had any effect on sensorium.
We had few successes in giving drugs to change mood, but
we had many successes by stopping drugs that either we or,
more commonly, others had started.

The expected number of newly developed diseases was
seen. There were two carcinomas of the stomach, two of the
colon, and of the bladder. We found one or two carinomas
of the breast each year and several unexplained upper
gastrointestinal hemorrhages. Basal cell carcinomas of
the skin were seen frequently. Chronic arthritis, collapsed
vertebrae from osteoporosis, cystitis, constipation,
hemorrhoids, dermatitis, upper respiratory infection,
stroke, broken hips, blindness, deafness, glaucoma, phleti-
tis, thrush, diabetes, hypertension, dependent edema from
immobility, and dry eyes and mouth were common.

Conventional medical diagnoses were of little help in
care of these people. If we couldn't change the functional
state, then making a precise definition of the medical
diseases that lead to senility, inability to walk, blindness, deafness. incontinence, and vertigo was irrelevant.
I only needed that amount of information which let me know
medical science had nothing to offer. A functional
classification was used instead of usual medical terms.

Those people who have lost independence and see
nothing in front of them except a further loss of independence are apt to be unhappy. The staff picked this up
and reported to me they were depressed and would suggest
that a psychiatrist might be helpful. The average psychiatrist doesn't want to invest a large amount of time in a
person with a failing memory, and he gives some drug that
decreases alertness of the patient. The results are usually
poor. We had many more unhappy than depressed people. More
attention to the patient from the staff and family was much
more useful than drugs. A glass of warm milk from a kind
person is a potent drug.

These persons were an interesting group because they
showed no progression in conditions. Our diabetics on
insulin did not develop retinitis or nephritis; our
hypertensive population had strokes in about the same proportion as our normotensive people. Our diabetic patients
with high blood sugars, but no urinary sugar, behaved like
our nondiabetic population. A person aged 80 does not die
of diseases that kill before 79!

We treated acute infections promptly with ampicillin,
tetracycline, or erythromycin. Nurses were instructed to
start the antibiotic whenever oral temperature exceeded
100°F, mental state of the patients changed, blood pressure

fell, or respirations increased. In the majority, cause of
symptoms was viral and antibiotics were stopped in 12 to 36
hours. We adopted this protocol because elderly persons
deteriorate quickly with infection and they may not make a
functional recovery even though organisms have been eliminated by the antibiotic given later in the course of illness.

Symptomatic acute cystitis was treated with chemotherapy and antibiotics when organisms were visible in a centrifuged urine and occasionally when white cells alone were
present. If symptoms subsided, treatment was continued for
2-3 weeks and the urine was examined before stopping treatment. If the urine was clear, treatment was stopped and
the urine reexamined seven days later. If organisms had
recurred, we retreated for a longer period of time. In my
three and a half years, urine was never cultured. We were
dealing with benign recurrent cystitis and not overwhelming
infection referred to in a medical center.

We did not obtain x-rays when we knew they would not
change our treatment. We x-rayed no joints. I cared for
12 collapsed vertebrae, which ran a typical course without
obtaining spine films. We would have acted differently if
the course had not been benign or if there were signs to
alert us to the presence of acute infection or a painful
neoplasm.

Hypertension was rarely treated. Many persons came to
the home on antihypertensive medication, and, if they wished,
we continued it. The problem of falling was much more
troublesome than strokes, and since I saw no real difference
in this population between hypertensive population and
nomotensive population, I usually held my hand. I'm not
defending this course of action; I'm just telling what I did.

When an acute condition capable of being helped by
medicine arose in a nondemented patient, the patient was
transferred to Duke Hospital, where we were able to control
the situation and prevent overdiagnosis and overtreatment.
When time for dying came, our families wished their relative
to die in the home without intravenous fluids, tubes in
mouth and trachea, or intravenous pacemakers. Many of my
people had my promise that they would be allowed to die
in the home in this way. When time for dying had come I
did nothing medically, with the family's permission, except
to prevent pain. If pneumonia developed, I gave no
antibiotics.

I was responsible for all aspects of medical care in
the home. An able physician's associate (our term for
physician's assistant) worked in the home for three-fourths
of her time and spent one-fourth as instructor in the Duke
PA program. She was administratively responsible to me and
not to the chief of nursing service. As expected, she
became as expert as I in handling all common problems in the
home. When an unusual problem came up, she recognized that

it was different and promptly called me. She did better
than I in the role of a friend and, in time, many persons
requested her services, knowing I would be summoned if
needed.

We gave support to the chief nurse and her staff and
took part in in-house training problems. My chief job was
to assure the staff that medicine had nothing further to
offer but nursing skill had much to offer.

We emphasized the role of the nursing staff as "caring
for human beings" and minimized the role of nurse as a
technician. In the technical role, neither the nurse nor
the doctor had much to offer. In the "caring role," the
nurse was irreplaceable. We worked with attendants to care
for patients who were dying and to treat them with feeling
until death occurred. I had to help them do this while they
knew I was doing nothing to prolong life.

We helped nurses decide how they would spend their time.
We invested little time in attempting to heal bed sores in
an unconscious patient who would never recover consciousness.
We merely kept down the odor. We invested much time in an
equally severe decubitus in a patient with deforming, crip-
pling arthritis and a clear mind. We reassured the social
workers and activities director that they were doing well
and that no experts could do better.

I was the patient's advocate in that I was willing to
take risks to maintain independence provided I had backing
of the family. I was willing to have a picture on the wall
and an overstuffed chair that was hard to clean under if
those articles meant a great deal to the patient. Our role
was to help persons live and eventually die. It was not to
cure.

From this experience I have drawn the following conclusions:

1. In the years ahead, with husband and wife working,
old people will either die suddenly or die in homes for
elderly. Home care programs can delay the time of admission
to the home, but they cannot prevent it.

2. The home should be a place for living and dying,
and the major amount of money should be spent on amenities
for living in partial to complete dependence and not on
medical diagnostic procedures or drugs.

3. The majority of medical care can be given by a
physician's assistant. The role of the doctor is largely
supportive.

4. The nurse must be taught and paid for caring skills.
She must be willing to run a less tidy shop than she would
run in a unit devoted to helping people with medical
technology.

5. In-service training for aides should be continuous
and should be rewarded by appropriate increase in salary.

6. Payment by government and other third parties

should recognize social and living needs of the aging
population and make money saved by sensible care available
to increase amenities for graceful, dependent living.

Part VI

Rehabilitation

INTRODUCTION

Harold B. Haley

The elderly recover from illnesses sometimes completely,
often incompletely. This process is slow and may last a
long time with small increments of improvement. It is
important to periodically document their mental status,
their functional mobility, and the physiological function
of their various organ systems.

In the introductory paper William Reefe defines
rehabilitation and describes a favorite area of patient
care, "Joint Disease in the Elderly."

Maurice Schnell, in an extensive monograph, reviews
rehabilitation and outlines approaches and evaluation
techniques of patients. He describes the effects of brain
damage on the muscular-skeletal function, the importance
of walking and its evaluation, gait analysis, stroke
rehabilitation, and the relationships of visual status,
energy use, and mental attitude in rehabilitation. A
detailed explanation of various rehabilitation approaches
is given.

Linda Kessinger outlines responsibilities of a state
vocational rehabilitation agency and its programs. She
presents a case report that illustrates how such a program
operates.

Peggy David, a social worker in a spinal cord rehabilitation unit, prescribes programs for bringing the
family into patient care.

CHAPTER 31

IS JOINT DISEASE ALWAYS DUE TO OSTEOARTHRITIS?

William E. Reefe

Rehabilitation aims to correct deficiencies to a degree that will ultimately assure maximum independence within the limits of the patient's disability. Rehabilitation has three components: a philosophy, an objective, and a method. The philosophy is that even the most severely disabled patient has considerable physical and emotional reserve. The objective should be to create optimal health and social conditions if maximal restitution of the disabled and the chronically ill aged is to be achieved. The method is demonstrated by a variety of professionals who must contribute the knowledge and skill of their own particular specialty The medical contribution to this comprehensive activity is identified sometimes as restorative medicine, indicating that the physician primarily contributes his medical knowledge and skill to the total rehabilitation effort. While his primary contribution is clinical experience, he must be thoroughly familiar with the role of each team member and have the ability to coordinate their widely divergent functions.

My single objective is to get across to you that all joints that ache in people over 65 are not manifestations of osteoarthritis. Remembering this one point is a big start in looking at joint disease in the aged. We tend to think that when anyone has painful joints after age 60, the diagnosis must be osteoarthritis. In a study we did years ago in a city hospital setting at a time when tuberculos arthritis was said not to occur in patients over 50, we had eleven patients in a year. The average age was 68, and these people were primarily in nursing homes and homes for the aged in the District of Columbia where they did not get yearly chest x-rays and where they had a single swollen joint for as long as two years before any effort was made to diagnose it. This is an uncommon condition, but where we are going to see this kind of septic-arthritis in the aged. If you draw a bell curve, about 15% of the patients with rheumatoid arthritis will have the onset after the age of 60. This, too, is not widely appreciated, and it makes a big difference whether a patient has inflammatory joint disease versus osteoarthritis.

Other types of joint disease are common to the aged. Gout may begin in the 40's and 50's and recur in old age. Pseudogout, calcium pyrophosphate deposition disease or calcification of the cartelage, is another kind of acute polyarticular or monarticular arthritis that occurs primarily in people over age 65. Polymyalgia rheumatica

is rarely seen in people under age 65. Many people with the
onset of gout after age 60 have underlying malignancy:
solid tumors, hematologic disorders, and polycythemia vera.
All lead to increased serum uric acid and can cause the
onset of acute gout after age 60 or 65.

In patients with clubbing and joint effusion we must
think of hypertrophic pulmonary osteoarthripathy, usually
with a pulmonary malignancy. In patients with back pain,
particularly females, osteoporosis with compression fracture
must be thought of; in males, frequently multiple myeloma
or other metastatic disease. The list goes on and on.
All I would like to say is, don't take joint disease in
the elderly as being caused only by osteoarthritis.

CHAPTER 32

ACTIVE REHABILITATION OF THE AGED

Maurice D. Schnell

Since aging begins at the time of musculoskeletal maturity, rehabilitation measures are applicable to a wide spectrum of the adult population. Techniques useful in disease and functional impairment afflicting individuals in early adult life are equally applicable to patients suffering from chronic disease later in life.

Effective rehabilitative medicine is a careful evaluation of each patient through a highly coordinated interdisciplinary team for the purpose of establishing an accurate diagnosis and appropriate treatment. Of utmost importance is a careful assessment of mental status of the aged. Rehabilitation is an educational process. Patients must have the ability to retain and assimilate information in order to change their behavioral patterns. With a reduction in cerebral arterial blood supply, the aged may have an alteration in attention span, memory, and motivation for recovery.

Some individuals may have sustained brain damage secondary to a stroke. Different types of communication problems may result. Visual problems, hearing loss, and speech alterations may affect the individual's ability to participate in a rehabilitation program. When the dominant hemisphere is involved, the patient may demonstrate both receptive and expressive aphasia. Severe communication deficit inteferes with the patient's perception of written and verbal language as well as preventing his communicating his desires and needs to others.

Brain damage produces a variety of motor and sensory dysfunctions. The most impairing is a loss of balance in the sitting and standing positions. The execution of simple manual tasks may be impossible if the individual has a loss of body image or demonstrates serious perceptuomotor deficit. Self-care activities, such as bathing, feeding, dressing, grooming, toilet care and writing, are taken for granted by all of us until we suddenly are unable to perform these basic skills. The rehabilitative process focuses on retraining impaired individuals to perform these skills. Yet most patients are much more concerned about learning to walk again.

Walking involves relatively simple, semiautomatic types of motor skills. Therefore, the primitive reflex patterns often seen following brain damage may be controlled through training, bracing, and surgical reconstruction in order that the patient may develop independent walking.

Approximately 70% of stroke victims demonstrate an extensor reflex pattern of the involved lower extremity.

This pattern is characterized by extension of the hip, extension of the knee, plantar flexion of the ankle, and inversion of the foot. The remaining 30% develop a flexor pattern. These individuals demonstrate flexion of the hip, flexion of the knee, dorsiflexion of the ankle, and inversion of the foot. Although both of these patterns can be influenced by proper rehabilitative treatment, patients with the extensor pattern are more likely to achieve independent walking.

Brain damage and other neurological disease entities often produce spasticity in involved extremities. This uncontrolled increase in muscle tones can lead to dynamic or fixed joint deformities. As a result, the patient may develop angular deformities of the hip, knee, or ankle. There may be curling of the toes, which produces painful corns and calluses. The foot may be pulled into a tiptoe position, which makes it difficult to bear weight through the foot. Each of these deformities must be dealt with individually in order to remove functional barriers to walking.

The rehabilitation specialist must have a keen understanding of gait analysis. First, one must understand the normal alterations of walking patterns from infancy through senility. Interestingly, the pattern of an infant is very similar to that of the elderly individual. Both walk with a widened base of support with little flexion of the knee or hip. The individual tends to rock or oscillate from side to side. The individual may extend his upper extremities outward from the shoulder in order to provide additional balance. In many instances, the use of external support in the form of a walker, canes, or crutches may be necessary to compensate for the loss of balance.

By understanding the basic phases and components of normal gait, the clinician is able to detect deviations from expected walking patterns. An example would be an individual with Parkinson's disease who walks with considerable flexion of the trunk and neck. The body is held in a very rigid position without arm swing. Turning movements are made as a rigid unit. Since the patient has difficulty controlling his center of gravity, he walks with a rapid, shuffling gait.

The visual status of an individual may also have an impact on his walking capabilities. A loss of position sense and truncal balance may be compensated for by looking at the ground and watching the lower extremities. This form of visual feedback enables the impaired individual to improve his walking skills. Deterioration of vision virtually eliminates this useful compensatory mechanism.

The energy demands on elderly patients participating in fuctional retraining must not be overlooked. Multisystem disease often plagues the aged. The status of the heart, lungs, neurological system, and musculoskeletal

system plays an important role in functional goals set for
elderly patients.

More important is the mental attitude of the patient.
The presence of depression, resentment, despondency, or
hopelessness prevents the patient's participation in a
rehabilitation program. Through counseling by members of
the rehabilitation team, many temporary personality alterations may be alleviated.

Establishment of rehabilitation goals for elderly
patients must be based upon their desires and needs. Both
the socioeconomic background and life-style of the patient
must be considered in determining appropriate treatment
goals.

Since many elderly individuals still desire gainful
employment, we cannot overlook this factor in the rehabilitation process. Job evaluation, vocational placement, and
job retraining should be made available to appropriate older
candidates. If such patients are retired, they should have
opportunity to learn new avocations to add interest and
diversion to their life-styles.

In designing a rehabilitation program for an individual
who has suffered extensive neuromuscular impairment, the
rehabilitation team must establish treatment priorities.
Ranking high on the list is learning self-care activities.
Through the use of adaptive aids and special orthotic
devices, many functional activities can be performed by
the patient independently despite significant physical
impairments.

Transfer activities are an initial step toward increased
mobility for impaired individuals. Learning transfers to
and from the bed, chair, wheelchair, toilet, and car sub-
stantially increase the patient's functional potentials.

The inability of an individual to walk independently,
with or without external supportive devices, is not the end
of the world. Use of a manually powered or externally
powered wheelchair allows the individual to move about his
environment quite effectively. Through energy studies of
normal and abnormal gait, we have learned that a wheelchair
may be more efficient than trying to utilize a slow,
laborious ambulation pattern. New wheelchair designs, the
elimination of architectural barriers and more sophisticated
wheelchair-training techniques make the use of a wheelchair
more feasible and attractive.

Individuals who are considered candidates for walking
must first readapt to vertical positioning. Stabilization
of blood pressure and reinforcement of balance is achieved
through utilization of a tilt table. Next, the patient is
placed in parallel bars and given appropriate temporary
lower extremity braces to stabilize involved weight-bearing
joints.

Gradually, the patient may regain adequate balance,
coordination, and muscle strength to walk without braces or

external supportive devices (walker, crutches, or cane).
Yet many patients need some type of lower extremity brace
and external supportive device to walk safely and independently. The design of the brace depends upon muscle power
and control, joint mobility and stability, and sensory
function of the involved lower limb. Balance, truncal
control, hip muscle strength, and intact-position-sense of
the lower extremities determine the patient's need for an
external device.

Increasing dynamic deformities of either the upper or
lower extremities secondary to spasticity often cannot be
controlled or corrected by physical modalities. plaster
casts, or braces. Soft tissue and/or bone surgery offer
another means of overcoming physical barriers to functional
rehabilitation. Not only do these procedures allow correction of deformity, they may alleviate pain, reduce muscle
spasticity, increase muscle power, improve coordination,
and provide joint stability. Frequently, operative procedures do not eliminate the need for supplemental extremity
bracing, although they eliminate muscle spasticity, which
negates the effect of the brace. These procedures are as
applicable in the elderly patient as in younger individuals,
provided the surgical candidate has no medical contraindica-
tions to undergoing reconstructive surgery. All postopera-
tive patients must receive carefully designed and monitored
rehabilitation treatment in order to achieve maximum results
from their surgical procedures.

In the upper extremity, pain and limitation of motion
of a shoulder may be alleviated through release of subscap-
ularis and pectoris major and minor muscles. Persistent
flexion contracture of an elbow may be relieved through
neurectomy of the musculocutaneous nerve and lengthening
of the tendons of the brachialis and biceps muscles.
Flexion deformity of the wrist with an associated clenched
hand deformity may be approached from several directions:
a flexor slide of the wrist and finger flexors; individual
lengthening of wrist and finger flexors; transfer of
selected finger and wrist flexors to the extensors of
wrist and fingers; and combined fusion of the wrist and
selected joints of the digits with concomitant muscle
transfers. Because of the highly complex neurological
control required for smooth, coordinated function of the
upper extremity, predictability and expected results from
upper extremity surgery is sometimes disappointing. Procedures which alleviate pain and deformity are usually more
successful than those which attempt to regain more sophisticated upper extremity function.

In the lower extremity, operative procedures are more
successful in the distal part of the limb and become less
efficacious toward the hip. Tenotomy of the long toe
flexors relieves deformity and pain created by curling of
the toes. Dynamic equinovarus can be relieved by a

combination of soft tissue procedures including lengthening
of the Achilles tendon, transfer of the posterior tibial
tendon anterior to the medial malleolus, complete or split
transfer of the anterior tibial tendon to the third cunei-
form or cuboid and release of the long toe flexors. At the
knee, flexion deformity may be remedied by release or
transfer of the hamstring tendons combined with a possible
posterior capsulorrhaphy. Severe quadriceps spasticity may
be altered by the quadriceps plasty. Adduction deformity
of the hip is improved by selective tenotomy of the adductor
muscles and neurectomy of the anterior branch of the
obturator nerve.

In fixed, severe joint deformities, soft tissue surgery
alone may be ineffective in achieving the desired correction.
For example, in an individual with a severe flatfoot deformity secondary to destruction of multiple joints of the foot
as a result of rheumatoid arthritis, realignment of the foot
may be possible through surgical fusion of three major
joints of the foot. Postoperatively, the patient must
remain in a plaster cast for three to four months. Despite
the prolonged convalescent period, the relief of pain and
correction of the deformity far outweigh the negative features of reconstructive surgery. One of the prime requi-
sites to undertaking this type of major reconstructive
surgery is an adequate blood supply to the foot and leg.

Many elderly individuals develop vascular insufficiency
for a variety of medical reasons. Much vascular impairment
may not be amenable to vascular reconstruction. Thus, the
patient is faced with possible amputation of the involved
extremity. Ablative surgery is truly reconstructive surgery with its primary emphasis on preserving a functional
limb. With the aid of advanced diagnostic procedures and
modern amputation techniques, viable stumps can be obtained
at much more distal levels in the extremity. Consequently,
this results in greater limb function with concomitant
reduction in energy costs during walking.

Through use of plastic materials, incorporation of new
engineering concepts and better understanding of biomechan-
ics, the field of prosthetics (artificial limbs) has been
markedly upgraded and expanded. From redesign of special
footwear for the partial foot amputee to complex, externally powered prostheses for high upper extremity amputees,
the expectation of gaining extremity function following an
amputation is greater today. Although the body-powered
prosthesis is still the hallmark of devices for amputees,
specific functional skills have only been achieved in
multimembral amputees through the use of myoelectric or
carbon dioxide driven artificial limbs.

Orthotics (braces) is another field which has had a
dramatic change through utilization of plastic materials.

Plastic braces may be molded by a vacuum system and lined with plastic foams to distribute pressure evenly over body surfaces, even in individuals with complete loss of skin sensation. The weight of braces often can be reduced and hygienic care of plastic braces is simpler.

Braces can be divided into two general categories: static and dynamic. Static braces may be used to hold limbs in desired positions of function, to present the formation of fixed deformities, or to add stability to weakened joints. In addition, following correction of joint deformities, such braces may maintain correction achieved either through serial casting or surgical intervention. This type of brace may be illustrated by finger splints, wrist and hand positional splints, knee cylinder splints for immobilizing the knee, and molded plastic anklets to eliminate all ankle motion.

Dynamic braces apply a force against a limb in order to enhance weakened muscular function to overcome muscle spasticity or to correct early joint deformities. These objectives may be achieved through the viscosity of plastic material used in the brace, power applied through rubber bands, springs, harnessed body power, or application of external power such as electricity or carbon dioxide.

Dynamic braces may be subdivided into several categories. A number of these devices depend on the viscosity of the plastic material to slowly alter malposition or deformity of the involved limb. The use of a plastic elbow-forearm splint in order to hold the hand and wrist in position of pronation is one such example.

Harnessing of body power to drive an orthotic device is another subcategory. The reciprocating wrist orthosis which is driven by intact radial wrist extensors or the elevation of a paralyzed forearm through use of the opposite shoulder muscles illustrates this type of dynamic brace system.

Reciprocating wrist orthoses may be operated by electrical motors or carbon dioxide gas, thus creating another more complex subdivision of dynamic braces. A less complicated subcategory is illustrated by Bunnell hand splints which are powered by rubber bands.

Control of the amount of motion in a joint with resultant forces being applied to joints immediately adjacent to the brace, such as in the double upright, bichannel adjustable short leg brace with a proximal patellar tendon bearing shell, represents another type of dynamic bracing.

Occasionally certain braces incorporate features rarely expected in either dynamic or static braces. Polypropolene ankle-foot orthosis serves to position the foot and ankle through the relative rigidity of the brace while viscosity and flexibility of the plastic material provide relatively weak dynamic force in lifting the foot during walking.

Use of electrotherapy and biofeedback is becoming increasingly popular in rehabilitation medicine. Through transcutaneous electrical nerve stimulation, chronic pain may be modified or eliminated without incorporating invasive techniques such as injection or operative procedures. Electromyographic techniques, such as insertion of small needle electrodes into paralyzed muscle, have aided patients in relearning functional control of paralyzed limbs through auditory and visual feedback.

One of the applications of functional electrical stimulation and biofeedback has been the development of portable systems for mechanically stimulating paralyzed muscles during walking. Surface electrical stimulators provide appropriate electrical stimulation to selected muscles via foot switches. Unfortunately, the necessity of multiple wires and the attachment of a battery pack to the waist are definite disadvantages to this system. Another system provides a surgically implanted electrode over the appropriate muscle which is controlled by amplified radio signal, thus eliminating the connecting wires and surface electrodes.

Although these systems have shown some promise, they have many operative problems. Often the muscle fatigues with repetitive stimulation and the benefits of the system are partially or totally lost. Furthermore, magnitude of electrical stimulus necessary to get a desired contraction of the muscle may exceed the patient's skin pain tolerance. These systems have frequent mechanical breakdowns and currently should be viewed as largely experimental.

In summary, the older individual should be carefully evaluated and considered for all available rehabilitative techniques. No pretreatment bias should prevent these patients from having every opportunity to regain the highest possible functional recovery.

CHAPTER 33

VIRGINIA DEPARTMENT OF REHABILITATIVE SERVICES

Linda Kessinger

As a specialized rehabilitation counselor for Virginia
Department of Rehabilitative Services, my goal is to assist
a client in reaching his fullest usefulness. To reach this
goal, it is necessary to tap all possible resources either
within an individual client or within an individual community. For 50 years the Department of Vocational Rehabilitation has assisted individuals in overcoming handicaps that
prevented them from establishing and achieving vocational
goals and adjusting to a work-oriented society. Our department has not worked with the aging or with those considered
too old for the labor market. Although our agency is not
set up for this labor force, this does not mean it presently
excludes elderly persons. Our society projects an image of
retirement at age 65. However, many age-65 individuals want
to continue working and our agency is now trying to help
them find employment.

For example, one of our clients, an age-65 self-sup-
porting farmer receiving a social security retirement pension
had a farm accident resulting in an incomplete paraplegia.
While receiving treatment at our spinal cord injury project,
we explored all of his financial assistance possibilities,
such as Medicare and Veterans benefits. Then our department
assisted with hospitalization cost and with further rehabilitation at Woodrow WilsonRehabilitation Center. Our trained
team visited his farm to assess the architectural, vocational,
and social barriers and find ways to dissolve them. We
educated his 73-year old sister regarding the
problems that paraplegics encounter. Then we provided
supportive counseling for his own disability and at the time
of his brother's death. Because of the incompleteness of
his injury, our physical restoration services helped him to
become ambulatory on rough terrain with a walker and around
his home with a cane. He is now helping his sister manage
their farm. This case history is similar to what our agency
has done and is now doing for our clients.

Now the legislature has modified our objectives. Something new and exciting for all disabled citizens of Virginia
and those in health-related professions has occurred. House
Bill 284 was signed by Governor Dalton. Effective July 7,
1978, this bill changed the name of the Virginia Department
of Rehabilitation Services to the Virginia Department of
Rehabilitative Services. The law allowed counselors to
serve disabled individuals without vocational goals, giving
them improved capability of self-care and enhancing their
family and their community involvement, thus fitting into

the agency's new goal of rehabilitation for independent
daily living.

The Department of Rehabilitative Services will be
developing and analyzing information on needs of the state's
disabled citizens. They will develop plans, policies, and
programs for providing services to those who need them, even
though they are unemployable. They will be providing services to prepare individuals for a useful and productive
life whether that be self-sufficiency or just a better sense
of well-being. Hopefully, money will be appropriated for
this new program. Our basic philosophy is changing, and we
are studying and are eager to learn about needs of our disabled citizens.

You who are working with the aged must write our
office and let us know the needs of the aged, and make
recommendations and inform us about the kinds of programs
that are needed.

CHAPTER 34

SPINAL CORD INJURY PATIENTS: EDUCATION OF THE FAMILY

Peggy David

In a rehabilitation setting or in an extended care facility,
our goal is to return a client to his home community. The
social worker's role, along with other team members, is to
keep that goal in mind from the beginning. We have a wide
variety of team members, but a crucial and often overlooked
team member is a family member. With our current emphasis
on deinstitutionalization, we must remember as we try to
transition people back to their homes from rehabilitation
settings or extended care facilities that we are asking the
family members to replace all of the professional team
members. It is a big task to ask a family to be occupational therapist (OT), physical therapist (PT), doctor,
nurse, nutritionist, and counselor to their family member.
    In the spinal cord injury project at the University of
Virginia Medical Center, the Department of Rehabilitation
Services established an acute care and rehabilitation program for the newly cord injured and provides a training and
education program for the family. Our results have been
interesting and may provide insights for similar programs.
As a social worker for spinal cord injury projects, my
clients are strictly spinal cord injured, but that doesn't
exclude other disabilities for which we now have a full
range of services. The spinal cord injured people eligible
for our project are Virginia residents, clients of Department of Rehabilitation Services, traumatically injured as
the result of car accidents, falls, or whatever, and not
disease entities, and must be at least fifteen years of
age. There is no upper age limit, so we do serve some
elderly persons. Most who come through our spinal cord
injury program at the Towers Unit of the University of
Virginia Medical Center go on to Woodrow Wilson Rehabilitation Center.
    When an individual is admitted, his family is told
about our program and our services. At that time we
emphasize that they are team members, although they may
come from a great distance. We give them a packet of
information they can take home. They read booklets on
spinal cord injuries, medical implications, and social
services that might be available to them. We try to
establish a date for the family to come back to a family
education session where they can sit down and meet with
our whole team. We explain their relative's rehabilitation
program, what is being done in OT and PT, and try to give
the family a realistic idea of what their future will be
like when the patient returns home. Any and all questions

are answered. Different families have different questions
and priorities. Then we arrange with them to come back for
a training day called a "touching day." We physically show
them how to help their family member and what they can do.
We take into consideration the health of other family
members. We interview the critical family member, the one
who will be doing the most with the individual. Part of
their training is to learn how to do such things as bowel
and bladder care. Also, we give them booklets showing such
things as patient positioning. We encourage patients to go
home on weekend passes or out for the afternoon or evening
and then come back.

In the past four and one-years we have worked with 290
patients. Approximately ten of their families did not come
for a family education session. Some relatives were out
of the state. One man couldn't identify any family member
or maybe they didn't want to identify him. Some of those
ten did come for training for the sit-down sessions. Of
the population that we have served, half are quadraplegic
and half are paraplegic. We are talking about more dependent individuals. As more people survive cervical spinal
cord injuries, there will be a need for more adaptive
devices.

Of the 290 individuals who went through our program, 24
were over 50 years of age. Of those 290 people who completed
their rehabilitation, only eight, or 3% went to an extended
care facility. Of those going to an extended care facility,
two were over age fifty. We believe that our family education program helps to make a significant difference in the
transition from institution to community and if you include
family members the transition is easier. You can't call the
family up on the day you want them to bring their relative
home. You have to begin at the beginning.

Part VII

Programs to Improve Health Care of the Elderly

The Veterans Administration as an Example

INTRODUCTION

Harold B. Haley

This book has emphasized societal, home, and long-term care, with little emphasis on hospital care. The Veterans Administration is developing national programs to help meet the needs of elderly veterans. In this section we look at how such national programs are currently being applied in one hospital with emphasis on admission units and their functions in patient assessment and placement.

Philip Fogg introduces the subject by outlining the principles underlying his managerial viewpoint in his hospital.

Ralph Goldman's third paper looks at institutional and noninstitutional extended care with analysis of costs and major factors controlling patient care in different settings.

David Walthall documents the recent history and increasing government and Veterans Administration roles in developing multilevel comprehensive care programs for the elderly. The importance of building education units for this purpose is emphasized.

William Reefe reviews some of the philosophy, problems, and procedures in establishing a new geriatric admission and evaluation unit in a large hospital.

CHAPTER 35

A Veterans Administration Hospital and Its Philosophy

Philip J. Fogg

Because people live under various conditions of temperature,
diet, sanitation, and other environmental influences and
because they have diverse genetic makeups, an adequate picture of the fundamental nature of human aging has not completely emerged from clinical findings, family records, and
vital statistics. Myths that all people over age 65 are
alike or that an older person is cute and should be treated
as a child must go. Important pseudo impairment derived
from apathy and lack of meaningful personal relationships
may imitate dementia or an organic brain syndrome that does
not, in reality, exist. Losses of position and social structure, economic status, and decline in interpersonal relationships and support often lead to withdrawal and depression.
Human closeness is an excellent antidote. When one gets
older it is often more difficult to make friends and self-
defeating defenses must be recognized by those treating these
older people. The older population is increasing in size,
whereas proportionately the younger generation is declining
in numbers. The anticipated population
States by the year 2050 is approximately 57%, that of the
older population is anticipated at about 125%. Therefore,
it is timely that society has taken up the problems of aging
and all its facets. The Veterans Administration is doing so.
 Over the last decade the Salem Veterans Administration
Medical Center (V.A.M.C.) has come from an 1,800-bed psychiatric facility to a modern hospital of about 900 beds
(including the 100-bed Nursing Home Unit). Over 300 beds
are mainly for elderly long-term patients. With the cooperation of management and the medical service, an internist
qualified in geriatrics and interested in the care of the
elderly was employed. One large building has been renovated;
two others have been approved for future alterations.
Living quarters have been improved. A multidisciplinary team
has planned for a 40-bed palliative unit (modified Hospice)
for an evaluation, direct admission, work-up, difficult medical rehabilitation problem unit, a psychiatric medically
infirm unit, and general geriatric units. Our Nursing Home
Care Unit houses patients of varying degrees of disability.
the V.A.M.C. has follow-up procedures on all patients from
acute care to discharge and follow-up in the community.
Nurse Practitioners are utilized for each unit. More social
workers, physicians for each two units, rehabilitation
specialists, such as corrective therapy and occupational
therapy on the unit itself, and physical therapy visits on
the ward will be available.

CHAPTER 36

INSTITUTIONAL AND NONINSTITUTIONAL CARE OF THE AGED

Ralph Goldman

There is a gap between the time that the patient is discharged, is no longer appropriately a hospital patient, and
the time that the patient comes back to the office or the
clinic. How can we close this gap? We can do so by using
what can be called institutional extended care and noninstitutional extended care. Institutional extended care includes
nursing homes, intermediate care facilities, and some forms
of homes for the aged. The other alternative--the home
alternative--requres certain reinforcements that have
attracted much public interest. De-institutionalization in
most cases must be discharged to a home. If an individual
does not have a home, we then must seek a surrogate home.
Some of the determinants. some of the factors with which we
have to wrestle, are largely the development of facilities
and personnel and resources to meet these needs.

The Veterans Administration has now changed the names
of its hospitals to medical centers. We are now at a high
level of technology both in equipment and personnel. It is
rational to focus such technology in the medical center.
In the past we always thought of placing patients in the
medical center--in the hospital--in order to utilize these
facilities. This is not always appropriate. For example,
there are many older patients who have senile dementia in
whom we may want to rule out some overt organic cause such
as low pressure hydrocephalus. These patients don't have to
be hospitalized for CAT scanning. On the other hand, one who
has been in an automobile accident, is unconscious, and may
have an intracranial hemorrhage must be in the hospital for
scanning. There are many other examples, but the reason for
the medical center is the availability of this high level
technology for both inpatients and outpatients.

If an individual does not need this level of technology
and does not need the frequent services of health professionals, alternatives are possible. The most common alternative is the nursing home, including skilled nursing
facility, intermediate care facility, and the unlicensed home.

Since 1963 the number of available nursing home care
beds has increased from less than 600,000 to about 1.4
million. They have more than doubled in a 15-year span.
There are more than a million people in these facilities,
more than in acute hospitals. The cost of all extended
care facilities nationally is only about 10 billion dollars,
as compared to 150 billion dollars for the rest of the health
care budget. In other words, the expanding needs for nursing
home care are not the major pressure on the health care

system. A more judicious use of acute care facilities could
provide for needed expansion in extended care without
increasing the overall budget. These factors need careful
examination.

Some factors must be considered in terms of planning
and extended care facilities. The utilization of United
States nursing homes by male patients is related to age (1).
In the "under 65 group" less than 1% of all individuals are
in nursing homes; over age-65 utilization jumps to 1.1%; in
the next decade it is 4%; and of men age 85 or older 18% are
now in nursing homes These fractions are even more dramatic
for women, of whom 6% are nursing home residents in the
75-85 decade, and 27% beyond age 85. Although only 5% of
the total population over age 65 is in nursing homes, or
in institutions at any one time, the risk of being in a
nursing home increases with age.

Dr. Wershow, who wrote on reality orientation for
gerontologists, has analyzed the last year in the lives of
persons who died over the age of 75 in Birmingham, Alabama.
His unpublished data noted that 80% were ambulatory and
fully functional within two months of death, and 60% within
a week or so--that only 5% were mentally confused or deteriorated, although many more became confused during the
terminal illness itself. If only 5% of the population at
any one time has severe intellectual deterioration, that
means that 19 of 20 do not. Therefore, since there are more
than 20,000,000 people over age 65, there are 1,000,000
people for whom we must provide the necessary resources.
The other 19,000,000 are obviously not going to require the
same resources at the same time.

To deinstitutionalize patients, the patients must meet
certain requirements. There must be evidence that the
option provides better quality of life. The option should
be less expensive, and the option must be medically,
socially, and economically feasible.

Why is there such a drastic increase in the number of
aged people in extended care facilities? First, there
is the geometric increase in the number of long-term disabilities. The risk of chronic disease increases with age,
paralleling the Gompertz curve. The scale is arithmetic
on the abscissa and geometric on the ordinate. Second,
nationally, only 8% of the female residents and 22% of the
male residents have spouses (2). Since women will outlive
their husbands by approximately a decade, the risk is
weighted toward women as opposed to men. The ability to
cope with the environment depends on an intact marriage.
As soon as the family unit is broken up, the risk of placement increases tremendously. In addition, few of these
residents had been living with other relatives prior to
placement. If there is a relative, the probability of
nursing home placement is relatively small until the last

few months before death. If that social support does not
exist, then the nursing home, or similar facility, becomes
an earlier imperative.

    Third, the condition that most increases the risk of
institutionalization is intellectual deterioration, which
becomes especially telling for those without family support.

    You have heard comments the last couple of days, and
have perhaps seen in the newspaper, about the General
Accounting Office report of home health care (3). Although
this report suggests that home health care is an economical
solution, the data support the opposite conclusion.

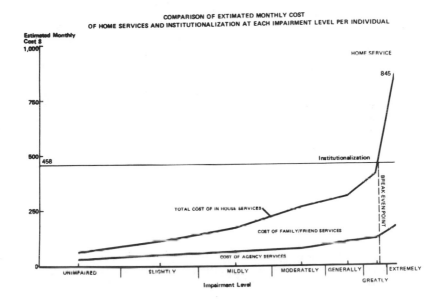

COMPARISON OF EXTIMATED MONTHLY COST
OF HOME SERVICES AND INSTITUTIONALIZATION AT EACH IMPAIRMENT LEVEL PER INDIVIDUAL

Figure 36.1

Comparison of estimated monthly cost of home services and
institutionalization at each impairment level per individual.

    Figure 36.1 was taken from that report, and you will
notice that if an individual is greatly impaired, the cost
of home health services is essentially the same as the cost
of institutionalization; in other words, in the most
severely incapacitated categories, it is a toss-up as to
which is the least expensive. The data also show that the
extremely impaired patients are 87% of the total population
in nursing homes. In addition, more than 90% of these
people, prior to being hospitalized or placed in an institution, were either living alone or living with people who
were not first-degree relatives. Thus, it is possible to

examine a community and identify the individuals who are at
risk of institutionalization. They make up that small segment of the geriatric population, with few alternatives,
who are least likely to be retained in the community.

On the other hand, many families caring for their aged
and infirm could use home health aids, but this would
increase rather than decrease public expenditure. There
are many costs, including social costs, that must be considered in planning alternatives to nursing home care.
First, there is the family loss of income of the person who
has become the caretaker. Second, there is often the loss
of a higher level of productivity to the community for a
lower one. Third, there is the loss of income tax to the
government that can be significant. Fourth, there is the
family exchange of a 40-hour work week of one member for
a 168-hour a week responsibility. When women were not in
the work force, we did not keep track of their hours nor
the monetary value of their services; we cannot discount
168 hours of service and responsibility now without assign-
ing it a value. Fifth, home care is labor inefficient. A
nursing home requires one person working 40 hours a week
for each person in the nursing home. Other alternatives,
such as a residential home, could provide a variety of protective and direct services for the equivalent of even less
labor. There are also the costs to the caretaker relief--
when the family wants to go to the theatre, to some social
function, or even to transact business.

Another factor has come out clearly. Many people who
are not in nursing homes would become eligible for home
health aids. We know already under Title XVIII and XX of
the Social Security Act and Title III of the Older Americans
Act that the Home Health Services have increased in the
last two years. The concept is important and necessary,
but in operation it will be directed to an essentially
different population.

A major issue is senile brain disease. There is much
emotion in this area. We are willing to accept that a
heart can age, become fibrotic and the patient can go into
congestive heart failure--and that this is one of the
manifestations of age and disease. But if something happens
to the brain, we want to believe that it is a social
phenomenon and it can be changed by social means.

Many studies indicate that there are significant changes
with age, and the neural tissue is subject to age-related
disease. It is known that neural cells are "postmitotic"
cells. Almost all brain cells are present at birth and
new ones do not form as the old are lost. We start out with
an estimated 12 billion, so we can lose a lot. There is
much of what we call redundancy built into the system, in
other words, we don't have to telephone directly from
Roanoke to San Francisco. The call can go through via New

York, St. Louis, or Dallas. Many alternate routes are
possible.
     Nerve cells deteriorate with age, and many of the
alternative transmission routes are lost. In viewing the
anatomic data it is surprising that function persists so
long, rather than the reverse. Yet most people function
almost as well at age 70 as they did at age 30. But make
no mistake, there are definite evidences of decrement in
reasoning power, in speed of response, in memory, and other
functions. Most of us learned what we had to know when we
were younger and we continue to use this knowledge reinforced
by experience. We are not learning new things as much as
we are applying old knowledge and modifying what we have
learned. New learning is possible, but it takes longer.
     We are faced inexorably with a certain number of
patients who have intellectual deficits with age. It is
important to make the correct diagnosis because management
can be very different for different cases. Acute brain
syndrome, most commonly manifested by delirium, frequently
isn't diagnosed, although the manifestations are clear. A
patient of 86 had a heart attack. Previously, he had been
intact with no evidence of intellectual deficit. He went
into the hospital and became completely disoriented and
delusional. As he recovered from the acute episode, he
became mentally clear again. This is a characteristic
episode. It is one of the false dementias. It has a rapid
onset in a matter of days or weeks, and a rapid offset in
most instances. It occurs most frequently in older people
because their margin of safety is less. It is usually
associated with conditions that reduce the amount of oxygen
to the brain--fever, heart failure, pneumonia, and drugs are
common causes. Most important is to treat the basic disease,
which is often life-threatening, and if that is treated
successfully, the patient usually will come back to normal
in a short period of time.
     The mentally regressed patient who needs long-term care
is the patient with organic brain disease of slow onset.
Average duration of symptoms for a group of patients that
were admitted for care was nearly three years. Generally,
someone who does not have a history of at least six months
should not be considered to have proved organic dementia.
These patients exist in large numbers, and they represent
several different conditions. The most common is Alzheimer's
Disease and Alzheimer-like dementia where there is a specific
pathologic change which can be quantitated with the amount of
intellectual deficit. It is a real entity and, unfortunately,
it is fairly common. In the Veteran's Administration we see
many organic dementias due to chronic alcoholism.
     Interestingly, relatively little dementia is due to
arteriosclerosis. This is now called multi-infarct dementia
in the new terminology.

There are other areas where pitfalls must be avoided. One consists of the patients who have been overmedicated and a group of patients who do have reversible dementias, such as low pressure hydrocephalus, or thyroid disease. These are not large in number. Of the patients who do not recover in a couple of months or so, less than 20% turn out not to have organic dementia. Organic dementias cause more than just a little bit of forgetfulness. Those of you who have been in nursing homes know the type of patient--the patient who can't remember his children's names, and often doesn't remember his own. There is no question about the dementia in these patients. Also, we must be careful that we are not dealing with depressed patients. These usually can be ruled out by physicians who are aware of these possibilities.

The frequency of all organic dementias progresses geometrically with age and is documented in the table for Japan, England and Denmark. This phenomenon is not localized, but seems to occur in every developed country where enough people reach old age.

Table 36.1. Prevalence of Chronic Brain Syndrome by Age

Age	Japan	England	Denmark
60-69	2.3	2.3*	0
70-79	5.9	3.9	1.9
80+	19.8	22.0	13.2
All ages	4.4	6.2	3.1

*65-69

Source: From Kay, D. W. K. "Epidemiological aspects of organic brain disease in the aged." In Aging and the Brain, C. M. Gaitz, New York: Plenum Press, 1978.

Figure 36.2 is a careful study from Sweden and shows cumulative, geometrically increasing risk.

The data are limited to Alzheimer-like dementia, and the cumulative risk of this one type of dementia increases to 5% by age 90. There also seems to be familial predisposition. The risk clearly increases with age, but affects only a minority of those who reach these advanced years.

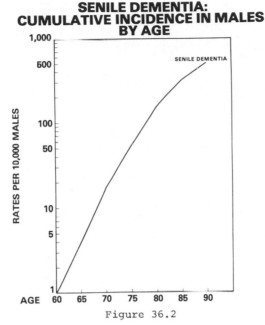

Figure 36.2

Senile demetia: cumulative incidence in males by age.
(From Larsson, T., T. Sjogren, and G. Jacobson: Senile
Dementia Acta Psych. Scand. Supplement 167, 1963.)

Table 36.2. Cumulative risk of senile dementia

Age	General population	First-degree relative
60	–	0.2
70	0.4	2.0
75	1.2	5.7
80	2.5	11.3
85	3.8	16.9
90	5.2	23.0

Source: From Larsson, T., et al. "Senile Dementia."
         Acta Psychiat. Scand. 39, Suppl. 167.

If we all lived to age 150 then we should all worry, but
that is not a problem now.
   The geometric increase in rate of nursing home placement with age is coupled with an increased association with
intellectual deficit, which rises above two-thirds at
advanced ages. Dementia is clearly a prime cause of institutional placement. The chronic brain syndrome is associated

with a high mortality. The impact of dementia on mortality
is obscured because the diagnosis does not appear on the
death certificate, and because the dementia may be the predisposing, rather than the actual, cause, which is often
pneumonia. But the risk of death is two to four times as
great for those with senile dementia as for the nonsenile
of the same age, otherwise at the same level of health.

These are the types of patients who present the
greatest problems for extended care. They are increasingly
old, they are increasingly likely to be intellectually
impaired, and they do not have social support in the form
of a closely related family. This is the problem, because
every day we must ask the question, "Can we deinstitutionalize, how many patients can we deinstitutionalize, what are
the alternatives to institutionalization?" It is a big
problem, and it is one which, for the first time, we are
addressing seriously.

Several years ago I went to give a lecture on physiologic changes with age. I turned on the television in the
hotel room to get the news and there was somebody talking
about physical conditioning. The question was asked, "How
do you know whether you should go out for jogging?" The
answer was, "First you should get a good medical check-up
and, second, you should find out what 85% of your maximum
heart rate is. You exercise at 85%, and as you get condi-
tioned you can increase the exercise and still maintain the
same heart rate." When I returned home I called a friend
who is a cardiologist interested in exercise physiology and
conditioning, and I asked him if he had a copy of the chart.
He sent me a brochure from the Heart Association, and guess
what? It went to age 65 and stopped. That was several
years ago. I didn't make a slide, so I wrote to him
recently and asked him to send me the material again. He
sent me updated material and now it goes to age 85. I think
that is the point of what's happening now.

When I was responsible for geriatrics and gerontology
in a medical school, one of my major responsibilities was
to make everyone who passed me in the hall think to himself,
"What have I done for geriatrics today?" I was not very
persuasive. It is twenty years later, and such persuasion
seems suddenly to have become much more acceptable. It may
be that eventually there will be an appropriate interest
in geriatrics, and this role of persuader will no longer be
necessary.

References

(1) U.S. Veterans Administration. "A Report on the Aging
     Veteran: Present and Future Medical Needs." Senate
     Committee Report no. 12, 95th Congress, 2d Session,
     January 5, 1978. Washington, D.C.: U.S. Government
     Printing Office, 1978.
(2) Zappolo, A. "Characteristics, Social Contacts and
     Activities of Nursing Home Residents. United States,
     1973-74 National Nursing Home Survey." Publication
     no. (HRA) 77-1778, Rockville, Md.: Department of
     Health, Education and Welfare, May 1977.
(3) Comptroller General of the United States. "Home
     Health--The Need for a National Policy to Better
     Provide for the Elderly." Washington, D.C.: U.S.
     Government Printing Office, 1978.

CHAPTER 37

VETERANS ADMINISTRATION PRIORITIES

IN GERIATRIC CARE AND EDUCATION

David B. Walthall III

This paper deals with the historical background of geriatrics and gerontology in the Veterans Administration (V.A.), the presidential and political implications for geriatrics, the V.A. Office of Academic Affairs' philosophical commitment, and the things the Office of Academic Affairs has done to implement these commitments.

As a country we started out late getting interested in geriatrics. Only after the White House Conference in 1971 was there any significant legislation. In 1972 the manpower grant legislation gave the Office of Academic Affairs the authority to make grants to medical schools, and some of those grants were made in geriatrics. In 1973 the V.A. Chief Medical Director, Dr. Jack Chase, identified geriatrics as a high priority area. In 1975 the Office of Extended Care, which Dr Goldman represents, was established. In 1976 our regional medical education centers were established, and in 1977 approximately 25% of our programs had a geriatric focus. In 1978 we began our geriatric fellowships, and the V.A. is now in the vanguard of the geriatric and gerontology movement around the country.

At a recent program on geriatrics/gerontology, Dennis Prager, from the Office of Science and Technology of the President, stated there are now approximately 23 million people over age 65, about 11% of the population. They now comprise about 17% of the electorate, so they are voting out of proportion to their numbers. In the five major states that have the most electoral votes, the aging population is more skewed. In the year 2000, 22% of the population will be geriatric. If the voting proportion stays out of proportion to the same degree, the elderly would be controlling one-third of the vote. By 1990 about two-thirds of all males over 65 will be veterans. That means that approximatel half, or 33%, will be veterans. What are the pragmatic consequences of these numbers on future legislation? Our economy may be smaller, and more and more emphasis is going to be placed legislatively on gerontology and geriatrics. Again, according to Dennis Prager, the president perceives that the high priority areas for agencies are alcoholism, rehabilitation, and aging. Alcoholism and rehabilitation also have a lot to do with gerontology.

The former Assistant Chief Medical Director, Dr. William Mayer, appointed a special assistant to coordinate all the geriatric programs occurring in the Office of

Academic Affairs. Dr. Donald Custis, the Chief Medical
Director and former Deputy Director of Academic Affairs,
has a strong personal interest in gerontology. In education
we like to decentralize control. We feel so strongly about
gerontology that we are not willing now to relinquish all
the control in gerontology education. We want to make sure
that a fair percentage of our budget does get spent on
gerontological programs. We have special management-by-
objective statements in our office that deal with gerontology.
The zero-based budget for the education and training section
had specific items in it for gerontology in the 1980 budget.
Our highest level decision package dealing with aging was
picked by the agency in preference to the lower levels of
funding, which demonstrates high agency priority in gerontology.
     What are the main things the Office of Academic Affairs
is doing now? We are trying to create multidisciplinary
teams with stipends and instructor support. While we don't
have any budget in 1979, we will probably take funds from
other programs. We have six fellowship programs and ten
fellows appointed now and we are selecting six more sites
and twelve more fellows for next year. This training program
is multidisciplinary in nature and interdisciplinary in focus.
     In the continuing education arena, our Office of Aca-
demic Affairs has had a national program in gerontology for
the past three years; we had a national meeting; we have
allowed participants to apply for a $2,500 continuing edu-
cation grant to be used in a geriatric program of their own
choosing at their own hospitals. We are having another
meeting combining most of the educational geriatric interests
in conjunction with a national gerontology meeting. Veterans Administration Regional Medical Education Centers are
being strongly encouraged to participate in gerontology.
Our centrally funded programs under the direction of Dr.
Goldman have a high priority at the V.A. Central Office
level.
     In summary, our belief is that there is a demonstrated
need. We are working toward meeting it.

CHAPTER 38

THE ESTABLISHMENT OF A NEW GERIATRIC

ADMISSION AND EVALUATION UNIT

William E. Reefe

My background as chief of medicine is unusual. My subspecialty is rheumatology, and I deal primarily with
outpatients and with aged people. I trained in physical
medicine and rehabilitation, as well as internal medicine,
and was in private practice for some 7 years. This led me
to various places like Hebrew Homes for the Aged and Blue
Plains, the District of Columbia's home for the aged. I
spent a year in the hospital with a chronic disease. This
gives me a little different slant on the subject than you
will find in most chiefs of medicine in academic institutions.

In our catchment area, the number of veterans over age
50 is projected to increase by 38% in 1980 and 130% in 1985.
This gives you some idea of the magnitude of our problem.

The extended care area is the only area in our Veterans
Administration Medical Center (V.A.M.C.) where we have a
waiting list. What are we doing about it? Dr. William Poe
came with us as chief of our long-term care section. This
has enabled us to give status to, and to bring education
and the educational opportunity into, geriatrics and long-
term care in our medical center. This is very important.
Dr. Poe comes to our morning report, the room is crowded
with medical students, residents, and staff, and they see
someone who is their peer taking care of the elderly. He
is able to answer questions as to why we did this and that
for this particular patient. We are trying to get the right
people involved. The rest is speculation.

To get the kind of people we need to work in geriatrics,
we must attract young people and give rewards to those who
have spent many years in it without recognition. We have
applied for a geriatrics fellowship program with the
Veterans Administration. If our application is not accepted,
we will go ahead with the fellowship program from other
funds.

We would like to begin with an admission ward. Instead
of transferring patients to the intermediate service, when
we are full on the acute medical service, we will ask Dr.
Poe to see a patient in consultation. Then Dr. Poe will
decide whether or not to accept the patient. This is an
important forward step. Hopefully, we will establish a
30-bed admission ward with a finite limit on the length of
time a patient can stay in this ward. On this ward Dr. Poe,
fellows, and other physicians will be taking care of patients.

There should be a rehabilitation nurse, a nurse practitioner interested in geriatrics, a medical social worker, and representatives from physical medicine and rehabilitation on this ward. Every patient who is admitted to our long-term care section would first be admitted to this unit. The team would see the patient upon admission and, within a few days, define goals for the patient. Ten beds would be available for those requiring intensive rehabilitation. At the end of 30, 45, or 60 days, whatever Dr. Poe feels is necessary, but it must be a finite period of time, this group would meet for the third or fourth time with the patient and his family and make a decision regarding goals for the patient. Then, if this is a chronic institutional patient for which we provide long-term care we will send the patient to a particular ward. If the goal is to return the patient to the family, that we will do. If it is to home care and nursing, if it is to a halfway house or to a nursing home in the community, we will proceed from there.

In addition, we would like to set up an outpatient clinic for the elderly in which Dr. Poe's ideas and methods of treating the elderly patients with dignity are carried out. Also, there should be enough staff so the physician taking care of these patients on the chronic long-term wards can follow these patients when they are transferred back to the acute medical service, or to the surgical service, and thus instruct these people on the acute services how the elderly should be managed. We would like to set up a home care program.

There are many things we don't know in the V.A. in the treatment of the elderly. For instance, how much physician input is necessary on a 50 bed long-term-care ward? What we are doing now, through the cooperation of the nursing service and our pioneer nurse practitioner, Jan Austin, is to have a nurse practitioner-run ward. How much physician input is necessary for that ward to function correctly? We would like to find out. We should do a retrospective study. What kinds of patients occupy these beds? All of these questions will direct ongoing research.

Part VIII

Clinical Miniproblems and Their Solutions

Edited by E. Gifford Ammermann

Introduction

Discussions in the conference sessions were practical and
thoughtful. Reporting of individual subjects is arranged
under the following headings:
    Women Veterans
    Prevention of Aging Disabilities
    Geriatric Education of Medical Students
    Access to Care
    Operation of Nursing Homes
    Details of Body Care (wheelchairs, decubiti, drainage,
        and cushions)
    "Patient" vs "Client"
    Nutrition
    Renal Problems
    Communication

CHAPTER 39

QUESTIONS AND ANSWERS

Potpourri of the Intriguing and the Practical

During the course of the 1978 Aging and Health Conference, there was opportunity for the participants to get answers to specific questions. These are grouped as to topic.

Women Veterans

Question 1: What preparation is the Veterans Administration making for the aging female veterans who are entitled to V.A. benefits? Many are now age 60 and will be applying for benefits in greater numbers as they become widows or retire.

Dr. William Reefe. When I came to the Salem Veterans Administration Medical Center (V.A.M.C.) seven years ago, we wanted to transfer a female patient from the acute medical service to a long-term care service. I was told, "We can't do that; we have only one big bathroom and we can't have men and women patients on the same floor." Since then we have renovated our long-term care units and now have many bathrooms for both sexes. Women are welcome on our long-term care floors. About 3% of our patient population are women veterans. I don't see why we should have any more difficulty treating women than men.

Dr. Ralph Goldman. Of 30,000,000 veterans, only 600,000 are women. Many of the older V.A. facilities. the barracks type, do not have private rooms or separate facilities, thus making it difficult to place women patients. With our current response to needs for patient privacy and other requirements, these facilities will be renovated Since more than 97% of American veterans are male, we are not being sexist in referring primarily to male statistics. Although we do so, we are planning to provide everything necessary for the women veterans who require treatment.

Prevention of Aging Disabilities

Question 2: Why is no attention being paid to the prevention of the physical and mental disabilities of aging?

Dr. Goldman. I heard an apt comment several years ago. Life was "nothing but a self-limited disease, ended by death." If one looks at aging as a pathologic process and wants a flip reponse, that is as good a definition as any. I believe, however, that much of what we call chronic disease in old age is actually a manifestation of the aging process.

In those disease processes that are easily preventable, we have prevented them. How many of you have seen a case of poliomyelitis in the past 15 years? Or a patient with tuberculosis? If there were as much tuberculosis today as in 1900 in Los Angeles County, there would be 15,000 deaths a year. There are approximately 60 deaths a year now, and these mainly in people who have immigrated from foreign lands. We can prevent or treat tuberculosis, and by and large it has been eliminated. Several years ago I prepared a text for public health and nursing students. One chapter was on nutrition. I tried to obtain recent pictures of patients with scurvy, beriberi, and pellagra. I could not find any. Old pictures or ones taken abroad were used. In summary, those diseases that we can prevent (or treat), we prevent (and treat) with remarkable speed.

Chronic disease poses a different problem. For example, educational weeks devoted to hypertension are supposed to cause people to become aware of this condition and, if present, have it treated. If we are to improve the prognosis in patients with hypertension, we must begin treating these patients at age 20, and perhaps by age 65 we will have improved their chances of surviving 45 years. We do not have a single effective treatment for hypertension that has been in use for more than 20 years. We do not know what the delayed effects of these drugs will be. It took us 50 years to discover that phenacetin caused kidney disease when taken chronically. We give many of our patients the benign drug hydrochlorothiazide, which decreases the excretion of calcium. Does hydrochlorothiazide keep the calcium in the bone or deposit it in the blood vessels? As we have been using it only since 1955, we do not know whether in 40 years we are going to pay for the protection from hypertension by producing more heart disease or some other calamity. This might be a problem, although I doubt it will be true for this drug.

Many chronic diseases have "risk factors." We do not have a long enough history or knowledge to know whether we are doing good or evil in controlling these risk factors. You may know the story of Tolbutamide, the oral diabetic drug. Fifteen years after its introduction the question arose. "Does it produce more heart disease without affecting the course of diabetes?" We still don't know, but strong evidence suggests this is the case.

In acute disease, treatment or preventative agents can be rapidly evaluated, and effective agents and procedures can rapidly be chosen. In chronic disease processes, evaluation takes many years. This time increases the difficulty and length of time needed to choose effective agents and/or procedures for control. The discovery of side effects, both good and bad, also takes much longer to discover. We are slowly learning and applying what we discover

but still have time to wait until we know what will be the
best answers.

Question 3: Is organic brain syndrome diagnosed very often
in diabetics?

Dr. Reefe. We see many patients with "arteriosclerotic
brain disease" in association with late onset diabetes.
This appears to be a common combination and, certainly,
patients with diabetes are as vulnerable, if not more so,
than any other member of the population.

Geriatric Education of Medical Students

Question 4: Are students receptive to the new emphasis on
geriatrics? They want hard facts, not soft philosophical
attitudes.

Dr. Richard Lindsay. The American Medical Student Association has been one of the leading forces prodding medical
schools to have curricular content dealing with geriatrics.
In our own institution, we have the same situation. How
does one get this emphasis into the curriculum?
     In reality, our students are extremely receptive. This
generation of medical students is an intelligent, caring
group. This caring attitude is also expressed in their
interest in geriatrics. They feel a greater need to be able
to take care of the elderly patient than many of our current
generation. The real challenge is to take their desire and
keep it alive and active. We must reach them in the early
stages of their medical careers before they develop the
negative attitude on aging that results from dealing with
the 5% elderly patient population that is hospitalized.

Dr. Daniel Mohler. As the questioner noted, students are
probably more interested in hard facts than in soft philosophical attitudes. One of the current thrusts in geriatrics is the generation of more facts: pieces of knowledge
that need to be imparted to our students in the area of
geriatrics. We hope to study the types of units mentioned
by Drs. Reefe and Lindsay. These units will be designed for
patient care and for doing patient-oriented research so that
we have hard facts to present to students.

Dr. Lindsay. One of the things that has helped to change
the attitudes some students might have had has been their
exposure on the medical service at the Salem Veterans
Administration Medical Center. For the past seven years
University of Virginia medical students have spent part of
their training in Roanoke. They recognize that Roanoke/Salem
patient population problems are the real world, and different

from those they have seen at the University. This experience gives them a certain amount of anxiety, and this
anxiety provokes their desire for information.

Access to Care

Question 5: How does an area, or region, go about getting
day care services?

Mrs. Pamela Lathrop. It depends on the area. The Area
Agency on Aging is required by federal law to keep a list of
services available for the elderly. If this agency cannot
answer specific questions about these services, they will
try to obtain them for you. If the local Area Agency on
Aging advises that a service is not currently available,
such as day care, they are required by federal law to tell
you about their two yearly public hearings. The first yearly
public hearing deals with need in the area and you can
request they provide the needed service. The second yearly
public hearing deals with budget decisions. Both of these
hearings are excellent opportunities to provide input into
the development of services and the area agencies are eager
to get an accurate assessment of the needs in their local
jurisdiction.

Question 6: What is the present status of information and
referral services for the elderly in southwest Virginia?

Mrs. Mary Elyn Lauth. "Information and Referral Services"
are designated as a required service. The Secretary for
Human Resources decided that a comprehensive information
and referral service would be provided by the welfare department and they are so funded. Federal law requires area
agencies to provide information and referral services for
the elderly. In addition, we have human service groupings
and various pilot programs beginning in parts of southwest
Virginia. In one county there is a "Community Services
Organization" that developed an "Information and Referral
Directory." An overall coordinated information and referral
directory is still uncoordinated and fragmented in southwest
Virginia, but there is a movement to coordinate on the state
level.

Mrs. Lathrop. A committee appointed by the secretary of
human resources is now working on developing a statewide
comprehensive information and referral system (I&R). There
will be regional information and referral centers in the
various HSA areas of this state. In addition to regional
I&R centers, there will be satellite centers in the regional
areas. If there is one central regional information and
referral center, it will have satellites in the various

areas. This is in the planning stage. Their draft document
of the statewide system will be discussed at public hearings.
When or where the statewide public hearings will be held, we
do not know. The State Department of Welfare is chairing
the committee and is a source of information.

Dr. Goldman. As both a physician and an administrator, it
strikes me that I&R is one of the fundamental issues that
we face. We have two problems. We have the nightmare of
patients who need certain services they aren't getting and,
on the other hand, we have an uncoordinated deluge of services. We are very primitive in our solutions. We want a
society in which there are multiple solutions to problems
and yet we don't want to have everything on a table of
organization; still, they must be available. We can do
this now with a computerized data bank. North Dakota has
worked out one not just for aging but for all social services
In North Dakota one can phone in, give certain information,
and obtain within 20 minutes a typed-out series of applications for things that the individual is eligible for, confirmed by the presentation of indicated documents and the
completion of the application. This is a computer age and
we need to develop these for the benefit of the needy. The
Veterans Administration is concerned. In our 172 hospitals
we have identified an I&R representative and we have had
nine training seminars in the use of I&R. These are the
essential first steps, but we are still in a "horse and
buggy age" in terms of implementation.

Mrs. Lauth. One comment about the North Dakota system.
Last summer I went to the University of Southern California
with people who are implementing the computerized data bank
in North Dakota. Some aspects of it are excellent and some
are less than grand. There is a case-management component
plugged into that system that says everybody has to go
through the same case management door, and this is presenting serious problems in the implementation of the system.
Also, there is a problem in the managing of people and in
getting them to the indicated resources.

Dr. Goldman. North Dakota does have problems. But I was
referring primarily, not to what seems to be a neat way of
checking in, but to actually getting out the data as to
where you can go.

Mrs. Lauth. This system is being widely touted on the
federal level as the solution to the uniform entry, one-
point entry system for everybody for all care--from welfare,
to aging, to health, etc. North Dakota has coordinated all
these agencies and all are going through the same door. All
you have to do is reach out and pick out all these things

because you have all the money there and it looks tremendous
on paper. The person goes through the uniform entry and we
take aging money, social service money, health money, and
all of these programs, and we suit the program to the person
and send them off to "Nirvana." It does not work that way.
When you talk to people who are trying to get the services
and the ones who are trying to assess the same people, it
is not as lovely as it seems. They did get waivers on certain eligibility requirements for some monies to allow them
greater flexibility, but this kind of case management is not
the total answer.

Question 7: Are home health aides on call 24 hours? What
is the earliest hour they will arrive at a home?

Mrs. Lauth. Yes, home health aides are on call 24 hours a
day. We had a case some weeks ago where a home health aide
went into a home and saved the life of someone who had taken
an overdose of medication. We go as early as necessary. We
try to keep our services within the average 8 A.M. to 5 P.M.,
five-days-a-week, but have been known to go into homes at
night, early in the morning, and on weekends. Each case is
evaluated individually, and we work with them and the demands
they present.

Question 8: Mr. Mays, do you work with counties without
ambulance service? Can you help an area to get this service started?

Mr. Frank Mays. Ambulance service is primarily voluntary in
this state and is provided through rescue squads. In the
future, lifesaving crews, or rescue squads, will find they
can no longer transport patients because they are being used
for more definitive patient care. We are pushing hard to
improve the linkage between free hospital care and emergency
care at the hospital site. We still do have a problem in
transporting incapacitated persons. There are private
ambulance services interested in providing this service.
Some local governments have an attitude that private ambulance services are only out to make a profit. If a private
ambulance service is to exist, there must be a charge
rendered for that transportation.

Question 9: I have a question that each person's presentation touched on, and that is transportation. I live in Mrs.
Lauth's district and drive to work each morning, approximately 46 miles up a mountain. I drive half of the way
looking into the sun and half of the way with the sun at my
back. This give you an idea of how you travel into the
mountains in the New River area. You don't go "as the crow
flies." What is being done about transportation?

Mrs. Lauth. We have sixteen vans taking people hither and yon. We take people in vans to programs. We also lend our vans to any elderly program free of charge. We ask them to provide a driver and gas. It is just a drop in the bucket. For over a year, as a member of a local transit study committee with the Virginia State Highway Department, we have studied our transportation problems. We have looked at federal and state funding. Do you know what we came up with? We will put another bus in Radford. At present we have two buses making a loop. We plan to change the loop and the buses will go off course. At least we will have something beyond the fixed route.

Operation of Nursing Homes

Question 10: In a profit-making institution, is there a rule of thumb or guideline when a full-time physical therapist becomes feasible? Is it at the point when 100, 200, or 300 beds are occupied? At what time did a full-time therapist become feasible in McVitty House? (McVitty House is an extended care facility and home for the elderly at Salem, Virginia.)

Mr. T. Stuart Payne. The daily average number of patients undergoing physical therapy in our 327-bed institution (McVitty House) varies from 18 to 24. A full-time physical therapist, as a permanent staff member, becomes feasible when at least 10 patients receive physical therapy daily. In working with seven nursing homes with approximately 105 patients, each had a half-time physical therapist. A part-time therapist can be used profitably in a 100-bed facility, especially with Medicare and Medicaid reimbursement.

Question 11: What is a good patient/volunteer ratio?

Mr. Payne. A one-to-one ratio is good because volunteers are not always present. We should have 300 volunteers who work twice a week, half a day. The volunteer in the long-term facility can do much by visiting with and making the patient feel a part of the community. That volunteer who is interested in the patient or resident is someone that many, many residents lack. We would like 50 to 75 volunteers in our institution on a daily basis, half in the morning and half in the afternoon.

Question 12: Briefly discuss the staffing patterns at McVitty House with particular reference to patient/staff ratios. How many people do you have to care for your 327 patients?

Mr. Payne. We have three floors with two wings on each
floor. Our staffing patterns are the same on the two wings;
however, on the floor that has 26 of its 50 beds certified
as being for skilled care, we try to maintain six aides, one
orderly, and two licensed nurses on the daylight shift. On
the evening shift, we have six aides, one orderly, and one
licensed nurse. On the night shift, one licensed nurse and
four aides are on duty. We do not have an orderly for
every wing on the night shift. We have one orderly for
every floor, which is three orderlies at night instead of
six that are on the other shifts. On the floor where we
have the more alert patients requiring less care, for the
7-3 shift, we never staff under two nurses, one orderly, and
four aides, and try to maintain five aides.

Dr. John Boyd. In speaking of staff/patient ratio, we not
only include those who attend the patients but count all
employees--roughtly, 327 employees as well as 327 patients.

Mr. Payne. Some of the employees are part-timers. For
example, our pharmacy is manned by three different phar-
macists. Each pharmacist works one or two days a week.
Included in this ratio are our yard, ground, and building
maintenance groups and our laundry and housekeeping groups.
They all affect patient care.

Question 13: What is your financial mix? What percent of
your total patient population is reimbursed by Medicaid?

Dr. Boyd. Between 65% and 75% of our patients are reimbursed
by Medicaid.

Question 14: With that ratio of Medicaid to total patients,
how are you compensated for the medical director's salary?
I assume he is a full-time physician.

Mr. Payne. Last year, Medicaid questioned us about administrative salaries being out of line. They were comparing
McVitty House, a 327-bed facility, with a 120-bed facility.
We were not penalized. Although overall administrative
salaries have been questioned, our medical director's salary
has never been questioned.

Question 15: With the difficulty some facilities have of
obtaining volunteers, do you think a public relations
specialist will provide more volunteers?

Dr. Boyd. We have employed a part-time public relations
man and have a staff member who is in charge of volunteers.
Our number of volunteers over the past three months has
increased. We hope it will snowball as we get people

interested and they tell their friends. This is often
the way it works.

Dr. William Poe. At Friendship Manor we had a very successful volunteer program. A delightful person, a minister's
wife must have convinced a number of ladies that their
salvation depended upon this form of service. We have over
a hundred volunteers who had a uniform or smock similar to
the Gray Ladies in the Red Cross. Get yourself a good pro-
moter and you will succeed in gaining volunteers.

Mr. Payne. Our director of volunteers, our activities
director, volunteers, and residents spent a day at our
largest local shopping mall soliciting volunteers and were
very successful.

Question 16: What constitutes skilled care as compared with
intermediate care? Sometimes even physicians, administrators, and nurses can't agree.

Dr. Boyd. Skilled care is defined as meeting the needs of
an individual who requires a service on a daily or hourly
basis by a registered nurse. Examples of skilled care
include large open wounds, patients requiring irrigation
of the urinary bladder several times a day, or patients
being tube fed and having problems with choking. A patient
requiring a hypodermic medication that requires the judgment
of a registered nurse as to the time that it should be given
is defined as needing skilled care. Occasionally, a physician will certify that a patient needs skilled care and the
insurance carrier will disagree. There is no clear answer
to this problem.

Question 17: How do you train your nursing assistants?

Mr. Payne. Our in-service training director trains all of
our nursing assistants in a three-week program that includes
classroom training and practice on the floor.

Question 18: Is the need for skilled-care beds really
minimal? In other words, why do nursing homes have so few
beds set aside for skilled care?

Mr Payne. The answer is minimal for McVitty House. We
have few patients who meet the criteria of "skilled care."
We have many more "intermediate" patients who require more
attention than some "skilled" care patients. Sometimes, our
resident patients should be classified "skilled" instead of
"intermediate." We do not reclassify them because of the
problems of moving of the patients and the amount of paperwork involved.

Dr. Boyd. We have 60 to 70 patients we could legitimately classify as "skilled" care patients. We carry them as "intermediate" care patients because they have skilled care where they are and we do not have the paperwork required if we put them on "skilled" care. There is no difference in reimbursement, so the "skilled" care patients are those from the hospital who truly require "skilled" care. They deserve their Medicare one hundred days or whatever part of it they remain on "skilled" care. In order to help these patients, we certify care as "skilled" and most patients we have on this status require "skilled" care. Medicare will only pay for "skilled" care.

Question 19: In connection with patients' rights. regulations, and restraints of patients, how are these ordered and how often do the orders for these have to be renewed?

Dr. Boyd. They are ordered by the physician.

Mr. Payne. We require a monthly review of orders and a renewal of orders for restraints. The order for "soft restraints as necessary" is written by the physician. Such an order is written on 75% of our patients. Our policy is to use restraints to a minimal degree. We have a disproportionate number of senile patients, patients with "advanced organic brain syndrome." A number of patients who do no harm wander around the halls, talk to whomever they can, and what not, but rather than restrain them, we let them walk. This is the best policy.

Question 20: What is your procedure for handling the investigations of possible patient abuse by staff? My experience has been that families are often suspicious of nursing assistants and are prone to blame them.

Mr. Payne. We go to the Director of Nursing and then to the nurse on the floor. We discuss thoroughly the complaint with the person accused of abusing a patient. We have never failed to follow up on a complaint. If the complaint is legitimate, and some are, then the abuser is dismissed.

Question 21: What are the criteria for admission to McVitty House?

Dr. Boyd. Criteria for admission are a completed application form and the submission of a history and physical examination form. In the Roanoke Valley we use a standard history and physical form that is reviewed by the Director of Nursing and myself. We avoid haphazard admissions such as when patients are dumped without provision for care or payment of bills. We require that two doctors agree to attend every patient, and we give our patients free choice of physicians.

Mr. Payne. The second criterion for admission is that some-one is responsible for financial arrangements. This is handled by our Director of Admissions before the resident is accepted.

Question 22: What guidelines are used that a patient may or should take care of his own room and surroundings? Is this regulated by law?

Dr. Poe. I don't believe guidelines are needed. People should be encouraged, not urged, not forced, but encouraged, to tidy up their own rooms. It is therapeutic for a fastidious old homemaker to tidy up her room and should be encouraged.

Mr. Payne. We don't have any guidelines or regulations. Very few homes do. We believe it is good therapy.

Question 23: What kind of staff have you planned for the newly opened home for adults at McVitty?

Mr. Payne. For 50 beds, we have planned one nurse on day-light shift seven days a week, one housekeeper, and two aides. On the afternoon shift, two aides, and on the night shift. two aides. That staffing does not include the food department.

Details of Body Care
(Wheelchairs, Decubiti, Drainage, and Cushions)

Following the series of questions on staffing in various types of homes and facilities for the elderly, questions dealing with rehabilitation and things to ease the physical discomforts of the elderly were raised.

Question 24: What type of wheelchair do you recommend for a patient with a CVA (cardiovascular accident)?

Ms. Karen Wolff. Most people are familiar with E&J (Everest and Jennings) chairs, which I recommend because they have many service centers. Other manufacturers of good wheelchairs include Rolls, InvaCare, and others. Almost all dealers have what is called a "one-arm chair." I do not favor the one-arm-drive chair because most patients with CVA's have difficulty in coordinating movement. They are frequently aphasic and cannot express their difficul-ties, and they may also have visual problems. If the patient is not careful, the one-arm-drive chair will drive him right into a wall. With this type of chair one is not able to

coordinate the two rims. Put the same patient into a regular
wheelchair with a removable footrest and you will find that he
can guide the chair with a two-arm drive. He manages with
his one good foot and his one good arm. You must support
the afflicted limb with a lapboard or with a trough. The
affected lower extremity must be on a footplate. The
elderly person does not have two or three years to learn
new patterns or techniques of mobility. If the patient's
mental status is satisfactory and there are no visual
problems, then the "one-arm-drive" chair can be considered.
Before you assign a one-arm chair to a patient, especially
one who is easily confused, you should have the experience
of trying one yourself.

Question 25. Are there any good regimens used for decubitus
ulcers other than applications of Betadine and saline?

Ms. Joanna Freskin. We do not have a universal solution
that is going to take care of all pressure sores. We have
tried remedies ranging from Maalox, heat lamps, Karaya
powder, alternating pressure mattresses, sandbags, everything from A to Z. Currently, we do not use any of the
above remedies except the "wet-to-dries" just to clean up
the area. We have managed to avoid most skin problems with
our patients. The vast majority of decubitus ulcers that
we get, we inherit from some other place. I can think of
only two patients with decubitus ulcers and that is because
we all work closely together to avoid these problems. If
any patient is the least bit red, all the nursing personnel
know about it within 15 minutes by our grapevine. The only
method that is going to clear up a pressure sore rapidly is
keeping the area clean and keeping the person off it as much
as possible.
     If the patient has several broken-down areas of skin,
we change his position; we "flip" him constantly. While
they are healing, we are also trying to increase the tolerance of the skin around the ulcer. We try to keep these
patients moving as much as possible, lying as short a time
as possible on any of these broken-down areas. It takes a
lot of nursing care. There is nothing easy and simple about
keeping these patients from having their skin break down,
and there is no simple, easy way to build them up again
quickly. It is a time-consuming process.

Question 26: When you use synthetic sheepskin, why do you
put it under the bottom sheet?

Ms. Freskin. We place the synthetic sheepskin under the
bottom sheet because this sheepskin makes patients sweat.
If it is placed under the sheet, the patient does not get
as uncomfortable.

Question 27: How do you convince the "powers that be" of the
advantages of leg bags (for the collection of urine)?

Ms. Freskin.   The approach we use is to raise the question,
How would you like to go around carrying a little plastic
bag with pee in it?   The leg bags have a floater valve at
the top that keeps the urine from flowing back into the
bladder.   This is a good sales point to bring up to the
epidemiologist or infection control officer.   Leg bags are
much more aesthetic.   We use them all of the time with our
patients.   Now we are using plastic, disposable leg bags.
We use them for one week and then discard them.   The disposable urine bags are easier to get from a medical supply
drugstore than regular ones and are cheaper for the patient.

Question 28:   Tell me about your use and selection of
cushions.

Ms. Martha Parkinson.   One cushion that is most acceptable
is called BBD, or "Bye, Bye, Decubiti."   It is inexpensive,
about $20.   It is an air-filled rubber cushion that can be
used in the bath tub when filled with water.   Being made of
rubber, it does not go through any lengthy drying process.
A big disadvantage is that it is difficult to transfer from.
If your patient has bad balance, he might be a little shaky.
     We do use various kinds of foam cushions.   Foam is
harder on sensitive skin than the BBD and it freezes up in
cold weather.   When a foam cushion gets wet, it takes a
longer time to dry.   We sometimes use the new foam developed
at Rancho Cimetics because we can custom-tailor these
cushions by cutting out places where patients are having
particular pressure problems.   The one problem with this
foam is that it wears out rapidly.   One patient just returned
with a similar cushion which wore out in six months.   Another
advantage of BBD is that they don't wear out, but they may
get holes.   In cases of extreme difficulty, we use a RoHo
priced at about $200.   Cushions are not the final answer.
No matter what kind of cushion a patient uses, you must
emphasize to them that they need to shift their weight.
We put our spinal cord patients on a regimented sitting
program in terms of hours that they are allowed up and the
time between shifting weight.   Weight shifting is important.

"Patient" vs "Client"

In the course of the discussion, a difference in terminology
arose that concerned many people.

Question 29:   I cannot reconcile your use of the term
 client" where I would use the term "patient."   Lawyers
have clients, doctors have patients, and teachers have
students.   Does your terminology make the patient or his
family happier or more successful in their role?

Ms. Peggy David. I tend to use the word "client" because, of all the team members here, I am not looking at the individual as a patient. To me, a patient implies that you are analyzing for pathology, assessing it, and planning to work out a treatment. I see myself as looking at the person and not as one who lays hands on the patient to treat. Therefore, I look at the individual as a client. My assessment is in terms of his or her strengths, such as personal and physical strengths, those in his family system, and those in his community. I usually don't deal with assessing weaker points, but rather in building from there and looking for strengths. "Patient" also implies more than the "laying on of hands," but implies a physical kind of treatment. This is my personal perspective. The question is interesting. We should note that all individuals at the Woodrow Wilson Rehabilitation Center are referred to as "students," even though they are in a total physical rehabilitation program. In terms of a rehabilitative philosophy, most people who come to a rehabilitation center are students on a philosophical level, even though they may physically be located in a medical center. The medical center would prefer to call them patients, but they are all present as students, as learners, and as relearners. We have scheduled classes every afternoon. "Students" is the best term. I do not believe this terminology has made anybody happier or more successful, but it has made me more comfortable with myself.

The term "client" is a historical term, the same as patient and student. "Client" has been the term used by the Division of Vocational Rehabilitation in each state for several decades.

For some, the word "patient" implies that there is hospitalization for some kind of sickness and that you are dealing with the person in a close, patient status. In rehabilitation, we do not want to prolong the idea that they are patients anymore but now they are a person again and are getting services. For some, they can best be seen as clients who are getting services in a different manner from the medical mode.

People don't appear to care one way or the other what you call them as long as you are doing a good job with and for them.

Nutrition

In viewing the elderly patient as a whole person, common concerns are sometimes overlooked. The most common experience of the elderly, and of those not elderly, is becoming hungry. The food they eat, the adequacy of it in terms of nutrition, taste, odor, warmth, and many other features are necessary to a rounded person. The next series of questions deals with with nutrition in the elderly.

Question 30: What are the most common problems of feeding
the elderly?

Mrs. Janet Austin. The most common problem is the fact
that food is often cold. Food comes a long distance from
the kitchen to the ward area. When food is brought to the
unit, personnel have to make sure that patients are prepared. Food is not delivered at a precise time every day,
and so the chance of all personnel being at the ward at
the right time is slim. We frequently have the problem of
spoon feeding 28-40 confused, elderly patients. The delivery
cart houses all of the patients' food and is cold when many
of them are served. We have been working on a solution to
the problem, approaching people who control funding, and
explaining the needs to them.

Mrs. Marilyn Donato. Cooking for 500 to 600 people is a
complex process. It is much easier to complain than to find
solutions. Even when solutions are found, there is expense
involved in trying to correct the problem. It should be a
continuing process in determining, discovering, and acting
on how to serve hot food hot. A microwave oven might solve
this problem.

Mrs. Austin. It would be informative to have an unannounced
sit-down dinner, for example, on a ward area where trays are
taken directly out of the food cart. Perhaps it would be a
low-salt diet or a lovely puree diet. Many things that we
prescribe are very difficult for patients to tolerate over
a long period of time. Trays are probably tasted and tested,
but we tend to forget the patient in the shuffle.

Question 31: What about the feasibility of having a pantry
to make coffee and simple meals in a nursing home, in addition to a centralized kitchen?

Mrs. Donato. It depends upon the physical layout of the
institution, its personnel, and facilities. Probably a
study would have to be done before it could be implemented,
and should be followed-up to determine how well it works.

Question 32: What about trace metals in the diet?

Dr. Sanford Ritchey. We know that zinc is required in a
well-balanced diet. Zinc has been recently discovered as
being particularly important in healing and in rapidly
growing younger people. In the older age group there is
a probability that low zinc intakes will affect the ability
of the individual to taste food. I am unaware of studies
indicating that there is a widespread zinc deficiency in
the elderly population. There may be a deficiency where

there is food restriction or poor food habits. It might
be useful at time of surgery to check plasma zinc levels.
However, as a routine practice serum zinc levels are probably not indicated. Zinc may improve the appetite of some
individuals. Zinc is only analyzed at occasional large
commercial medical laboratories and is not routinely available. Zinc and other micronutrients are present in larger
quantities than the average individual needs in a well-
balanced, well-rounded diet.

Foods that tend to be highest in zinc are meats such
as beef, pork, and liver. Fish tends to be low. Zinc
sulfate or zinc acetate could be tried as a short-term
supplement.

Dr. A. Sidney Barritt. Much is written today in the health
food faddist magazines promoting vitamins and the use of
excessive amounts of trace minerals. Nutritionists are
slowly getting the information we need, but these magazines
are promoting supplements without any real knowledge of
dosage. It will take several years before we have reliable
data as to the need for zinc, selenium, chromium, and other
trace metals. In the meantime, be skeptical about what
you read in some of the health food faddist magazines.

Question 33: Why do so many doctors order mechanical soft
diets when in many cases the person has been without teeth
a good number of years? This type of patient can eat
almost anything without having teeth, and yet we still
receive many diets for the unpalatable, mechanical soft
diet.

Dr. Barritt. I never do that. One reason is that Mrs.
Austin has corrected my bad habits. Why do physicians
often order these diets?

Dr. Ritchey. I believe it is because they don't think
about it.

Mrs. Austin. Right! Focus on what the patient can do.
Ask him what he can eat. Can he bite an apple without any
problem?

Question 34: After listening to the answer of the last
question, are you telling me that I can order a regular
diet for any of my edentulous patients?

Mrs. Austin. No! You have to ask your patients what they
can eat. There are some patients who are capable of eating
hard foods that you would not suspect. Diet histories are
very important. We need to know their likes, dislikes,
what they are able to eat, and what they are not able to eat.

Question 35: I try to take diet histories and find that everyone eats three meals a day. They say they have two eggs, ham, bacon, toast, and orange juice for breakfast. I look at them and know that is not what they are eating. Why don't I get the right information when I take diet histories?

Mrs. Donato. People try to convey a good impression of themselves when you are interviewing them concerning their diets. It takes time to establish rapport and to get the patient to tell you honestly what he or she is eating. I am not defending the physician, but he really does not have the time to into full detail of the small things that one learns about a patient's diet. If the nurse or dietitian finds that the mechanical soft diet is not working with the patient, it is easy to call the physician or to go ahead and make a recommendation.

Dr. Barritt. What I know and what I use to take diet histories, I learned from the dietitians. Their techniques in this field are much better than the ones we physicians learn and practice.

Question 36: Some people seldom eat before noon. These include both school children and elderly adults. I haven't yet figured out how they manage to live that way, and no amount of persuasion seems able to change them. They say, "We don't have time to eat breakfast." What should we do?

Mrs. Donato. If an adult feels that he can go through the day and function just as well whether he skips breakfast or whether he eats it, I do not tell him he must eat breakfast. It takes much time and it takes a commitment on the part of the individual before he can make any change in his diet. If a person feels well and can function efficiently when he misses breakfast and has a good lunch, then there is no real reason to attempt to get him to change his dietary habits and patterns.

Renal Problems

The next section focuses on people with renal problems, including the problems of high-cost technology and the day-to-day problems of managing patients.

Question 37: Many people complain about renal dialysis and transplantation because they believe that this is a halfway technology, it is expensive, and might be rendered obsolete. The only way to meet the problem of dialysis is to prevent the disease. On the basis of current data, what is the probability of future prevention of chronic renal failure?

Dr. Jorge Roman. I am not optimistic about the prevention of chronic renal failure. We might make some inroads, but the problem is here to stay. Until we have an effective health care system that addresses early hypertension, early immunological disease, and early genetically induced problems, we are not going to prevent chronic renal failure. Many of the issues are now serviced by halfway technologies. A halfway technology is better than no technology, but, at times, it is hard to be sure.

Question 38: What impact on prevention of renal failure is the early diagnosis and treatment of urinary tract infections?

Dr. Jay Gillenwater. I can give you data on the Calvin Kunin youngsters. Urinary tract infection constitutes somewhere from less than 10% to a maximum of 20% of the people who develop end-stage renal failure. The real problem is glomerulonephritis. Kunin, in 1959, surveyed approximately 14,500 children in the Charlottesville-Waynesboro area for the presence of bacteriuria. He found that 1.2% of the girls and 0.03% of the boys had asymptomatic bacteriuria. We are still following these youngsters. They are now in their 30's, and, statistically, they have a lower level of renal function than control patients. He had matched control pairs. For example, one little girl sat next to the patient and was the same age and race, but has normal clearances. Two of these children have lost kidneys to chronic pyelonephritis. The lowest creatinine clearance is in the low 40's. So far, there have been none with renal failure in this group.

Dr. Charles Schleupner. The known data agree with Dr. Gillenwater's comments. The incidence of renal or urinary tract infection leading to renal failure is quite low. Infection is not a major issue in the development of chronic renal failure. Infection becomes a complicated issue on top of other causes of renal failure. In the mid-1950s, Ed Cass proposed 100,000 organisms in the urine as the cutoff point indicating a significant infection. The internists, and I am an internist, bought this blindly. There was panic everywhere about organisms in the urine. On a few occasions when lecturing on surgical oliguria, I suggested that it might be wise to use retrograde catheters to be sure that the ureters had not been ligated. On two different occasions, people got up from the audience and castigated me for even suggesting the use of a catheter. Didn't I know that the catheter killed? In the early dialysis and transplantation era, it was believed that pyelonephritis caused uremia five time as frequently as did glomerulonephritis. Since we "knew" that glomerulonephritis accounted for 0.8 to 1% of all deaths, that made the frequency of renal failure around

5%. This would have caused astronmical problems in dialysis and transplantation. We now know that the frequency is relatively low. Approximately 55%-60% of patients under-going transplantation or dialysis have glomerulonephritis in one of its forms. Approximately one-fifth have pyeloneph-ritis. The ratio was one-fifth instead of five times as much pyelonephritis as glomerulonephritis in causing chronic renal failure. The remainder of patients have mainly con-genital anomalies, such as polycystic kidney. In spite of all our objectivity and demanding of scientific proof, we accepted the concept of bacteriuria as a major lethal com-ponent blindly, without realizing that bacteriuria is usually a secondary manifestation of some other underlying process. Unless the obstruction, stone, or anomaly is successfully treated, the infection cannot be.

Question 39: In southwest Virginia are there problems of access unmet needs, treatment, etc., in the problems of end-stage renal failure?

Dr. Roman. Now and in the immediate future, there will be unlimited access to dialysis and renal transplantation as long as society and medicine are willing to devote their time and effort. Access could be limited if Congress or the secretary of HEW withdrew funds supporting this small, but expensive, population group. Another possible road-block will come when our various hospital administrators and vice presidents for health affairs say, "Stop, we have more important things to do." In the short run, there will be unending increases in resources to which end stage renal patients can turn. It may be that society will state, "This is ridiculous; we can't afford these expenditures." Probably we are going to see the same application of resource expenditure to other health care areas, rather than a recanting of the expenditures and efforts now being expended in end-stage renal disease (ESRD). There is not any pattern of underserved needs in ESRD at the present time. Any underserved needs currently present are due to the failure of individual practitioners and patients in recognizing the availability of the services, rather than inaccessibility or lack of services.
     The only area currently being underserved systematically is that of prevention. The obvious way to solve a problem is to prevent it. Less than 1% of the money spent by the federal or state governments on ESRD and chronic dialysis is going into renal research. The current dialysis program spent 1.8 billion in 1977 and is expected to rise to 3 billion. The doctors are not charging the patients addi-tional money, because the fee has been set since 1968. The physicians still get the same fee per dialysis as they did in 1968. The increase of money is being spent on the

accumulating population now being served. Some in the
federal government believe it costs more money to do it;
it does, because more are being kept alive, not because
doctors or hospitals are receiving more.

One example of the vast reservoir of potential ESRD
patients is the numerous people with hypertension. Until
we are able to develop an acceptable, effective, responsive,
ongoing program to detect those people who have hypertension,
guide them to effective treatment, monitor their treatment,
and encourage their continued participation, we will have
no effective way of decreasing the pool of future patients
with end-stage renal disease.

Question 40: Please comment on the British experience with
their National Health Service. How do they select patients
for dialysis and transplantation?

Dr. Roman. They select patients in two ways. First, there
is a very heavy emphasis on home or self-dialysis. This
tends to eliminate the patient who is incapable of using
either modality. Secondly, there is an age limitation so
that individuals over age 60 find themselves ignored.

This topic is very hot in Britain now. The British
have put approximately 60 patients per million population
per year on dialysis, while in the United States we now
put 135 to 140 patients per million per year on dialysis.
Either the Americans are twice as likely to get ESRD or the
British are not accurately recording patient numbers. Mortality of those on home dialysis in Britain has climbed in
the past few years. This raises the questions: (1) Are
people being forced into home dialysis who are not capable
of doing it? (2) Are they ill-prepared to go into home
dialysis in order to cut costs?

Question 41: What is the place and the purpose of exercise
while on dialysis?

Dr. Roman. You have to differentiate between hemodialysis
and peritoneal dialysis, and also to consider the amount
of tubing a patient gets. A patient on hemodialysis has
5 feet of tubing from an arm, the usual place, to the kidney
machine. A patient on peritoneal dialysis has several feet
of tubing from the abdomen to the set of bottles. Previously, in the early stages of managing renal failure,
exercise was used as an anabolic stimulant to induce protein
synthesis and reduce muscle breakdown. With the degree of
dialysis now used, I don't believe it is important.

I do see one important psychological advantage to having
the patient move. Two of the big breakthroughs have been the
shortening of a hemodialysis session from 16 to 6 hours and
changing the patient's position from lying flat in a bed

to sitting up in a chair and even having the patient walk
around the kidney machine. I do not know if the change of
position or even the walking changes metabolism. I do know
it does change patient and staff attitude. A person who is
in a bed, attached to a kidney machine, looks awful and is
handled like a terminal patient. Someone in a chair watching
TV, playing cards or bingo, looks better and is handled like
a healthier patient.

We have had people on manual peritoneal cycles who have
not only been able to move around, but do normal housework.
One woman used to walk around with an IV pole and dialysis
bottles and do her normal household duties. One big advantage of chronic, ambulatory peritoneal dialysis (the 4 times
daily belly washer) is that the patient has normal activities
without limitations. I don't know if it modifies the
patient's metabolism, but it certainly helps their overall
feeling of well-being.

Question 42: Does the type of dialysis influence the
incidence of anemia, electrolyte changes, or osteoporosis?

Dr. Roman. Hemodialysis is accompanied by a slightly greater
degree of anemia than peritoneal dialysis. This is because
of the constant small blood loss in the dialysis lines. People on continuous ambulatory peritoneal dialysis (4 times a
day) improve their hematocrits when compared with that on
previous hemodialysis. Maybe the constant dialysis allows
for more efficient removal of an undertermined toxin that
depresses the bone marrow of the patient. Patients on hemodialysis have the worst anemia; those on intermittent peritoneal dialysis, an intermittent stage of anemia; and the
best blood picture is found in those on ambulatory peritoneal
dialysis.

In regard to bone disease and changes of calcium, the
data are scattered and uncertain. Some patients have
developed bone disease while having peritoneal dialysis.
These people tend to lose calcium, while people on hemodialysis tend to gain calcium. The reason is not yet known,
and is perhaps due to insufficient calcium in the dialysate
or may be linked to another problem. Another possible
explanation is diet. Patients on dialysis tend to lose
protein and, therefore, we tell them to eat a regular diet
which contains an excessive amount of protein. With the
increased protein they get an increased amount of potassium.
In order to prevent the buildup of potassium, we dialyze
without potassium in the dialysate and this solves that
problem. On a weekly basis, our patients on peritoneal
dialysis tend to follow their diets less closely than those
on hemodialysis. Thus they tend to gain weight more
rapidly on peritoneal dialysis than hemodialysis. This
weight is not tissue weight, it is water and fluids. In

removing the excess water and weight, we also remove
excess calcium.

Communication

Question 43: What effect does noise have on our hearing?

Dr. Roger Ruth. Many individuals have a hearing loss because
of environmental sounds, particularly industrial noise.
Regulatory agencies are now requiring individuals to wear
hearing protection devices on the job and to lower the overall ambient noise level. Anyone who works in a noisy
environment over a long period of time will experience some
hearing loss. The hearing loss from this damage as seen on
audiograms is similar to that seen in the presbyacusic
(elderly hard of hearing) patient. It is a high frequency
hearing loss with sparing of low frequency hearing. The high
frequency loss gives problems in speech discrimination. This
difficulty in discriminating speech is especially pronounced
in older patients who have worked for a long time in industry.

Dr. Robert Cantrell. Today, we recognize that noise does
affect us. The term "presbyacusis" is rapidly being replaced
with a newer term, "sociocusis." Sociocusis acknowledges
and refers to the combined effect on hearing of noise and of
physiological process of aging.

Question 44: In the older, mentally ill patient who does
not speak and has a hearing impairment, how can we evaluate
if he is having pain, and, if so, how much? In a similar
patient who is also blind, how can we evaluate the symptoms?

Mrs. Mary Wolanin. We all have certain survival needs, and
difficulties with these needs cause pain. You can evaluate
a list to see which one of the items could be causing the
patient distress. I would start with air. Is the patient
getting enough air? Is the air quality good enough so that
you yourself would be comfortable? Next, is the patient
dehydrated? Is he getting enough to eat? Does eating
distress him? How are his many mouth functions and his
swallowing? A patient with a speech problem frequently has
associated swallowing problems. Continue down the list of
problems that would personally cause you pain, continue
until you find his problem. The key is that we can use
ourselves as a model in looking at other human beings to
find out what causes them distress.

Question 45: Are there materials available to help the
families of aphasic adults to better understand their
communication problems?

Dr. Ruth. One source of information is the American Speech and Hearing Association, 10801 Rockville Pike, Rockville, Maryland 20852. It has material on communication problems with older persons who have had stroke, Parkinson's Disease, and other hearing problems, as well as patients who have had laryngectomies. There are also other sources of information to help these families.

Question 46: Phonemic regression has been carefully covered previously. Phonemic regression is the inability of a person to discriminate, to actually understand what is being said. A companion problem, recruitment, was barely mentioned. Recruitment needs to be emphasized, especially for physicians giving advice to patients regarding the fitting of hearing aids. We can determine audiologically the most comfortable loudness or listening level for a patient. People with presbyacusis, however, frequently have a narrowed range between the comfortable listening level and the uncomfortable loudness level.

Dr. Ruth. Presbyacusis involves damage to the cochlea, the eighth nerve, or other parts of the system. Peculiar to some types of inner ear damage, people experience problems with loudness tolerance. They have a hearing loss and you may have to shout in order for them to hear you. Their loudness perception increases rapidly. They become uncomfortable when they cannot tolerate the intensity of sound that people with normal hearing can. This compressed dynamic hearing range means the pressure between the very softest sound they can hear and the loudest sound they can tolerate comfortably has decreased. This becomes important in fitting a hearing aid on such an individual. The hearing aid simply amplifies sound. If you put a loud sound into a hearing aid and it makes it louder, the patient's hearing range is overextended causing further distortion, pain, and reduction of hearing discrimination.

Question 47: Mrs. Wolanin, are professional health care workers really responsible for the affectional needs of their elderly patients?

Mrs. Wolanin. In the acute, short-term intensive care unit, I am not sure that we are responsible for affectional needs. I would like to think that we would be sensitive to these needs and have some responsibility. In the long-term care of aged people, especially those who make their homes with us and those without families, the problem changes. When we view the problem critically, the questions change. Do we desire that the person live like a half-alive human being, or can we supply a little extra spark? An arm across the shoulders now and then, calling our patients by their

preferred names, asking them if they saw the baseball game
last night, or other personal concern, and looking at them
as we talk. This is the little bit of extra effort that
we can give that may make a person's day. It takes so
little to meet affectional needs that we have a strong
responsibility to consider and act on them.

Contributors

Index

CONTRIBUTORS

E. Gifford Ammermann, M.D.
Chief
Nuclear Medicine Service
Veterans Administration Medical Center
Salem, Virginia 24153
and Assistant Professor of Radiology and Pathology
University of Virginia School of Medicine
Dr. Ammermann obtained a medical degree and training in
Pathology at Northwestern University Medical School and
training in Nuclear Medicine at Oak Ridge, Tennessee.
Dr. Ammermann is chairman of the Radioisotope Committee
at the Salem Veterans Administration Medical Center and
member of many other hospital committees. He teaches water
safety and navigation as a member of the Roanoke Valley
Power Squadron.

Janet M. Austin, R.N.
Medical Nurse Practitioner
Veterans Administration Medical Center
Salem, Virginia 24153
Janet M. Austin is a graduate of the University of Rochester
nurse practitioner program. Currently, she is nurse administrator of an intermediate care unit (Mrs. Austin is changing
the attitudes of an interdisciplinary team of health care
professionals to view "aging as beautiful, if you look, act,
and care").

A. Sidney Barritt III, M.D.
Assistant Chief
Medical Service
Veterans Administration Medical Center
Salem, Virginia 24153
and
Assistant Professor of Internal Medicine
University of Virginia School of Medicine
Dr. Barritt obtained a medical degree at Cornell University
Medical College, his training in internal medicine at the
University of Virginia, and training in gastroenterology at
the Medical College of Virginia. As chairman of the Salem
Veteran's Administration Medical Center Nutrition Committee,
he is a consultant to all areas of the hospital and is
experienced in the special needs of the older patient.

John O. Boyd, Jr., M.D.
Medical Director
McVitty House, Inc.
Salem, Virginia 24153
Dr. Boyd was in general practice in Roanoke until 1967. A
former president of the Virginia Association of Family

Practitioners, Dr. Boyd served on the board of McVitty
House, Inc., a nursing home, for twenty years. In 1975
he joined their staff as full-time medical director.

James A. Bryan III, M.D.
Professor of Medicine
Department of Medicine and Hematology
University of North Carolina at Chapel Hill School of
  Medicine
Chapel Hill, North Carolina 27514
Two years at the Center for Disease Control, Public Health
Service and a career as a hematologist/oncologist in
teaching hospitals have made him aware that "health or
wholeness can be claimed by persons in all stages of life--
even those on the brink of death."

Robert W. Cantrell, M.D.
Fitz-Hugh Professor and Chairman
Department of Otolaryngology and Maxillofacial Surgery
University of Virginia School of Medicine
Charlottesville, Virginia 22908
Dr. Cantrell was chairman of the Department of Otolaryngology,
Naval Regional Medical Center, San Diego, California, before
assuming his present post. In 1974 he received the Harris
P. Mosher Award for excellence in clinical research for his
work on the effects of prolonged exposure to intermittent
noise. Dr. Cantrell has a keen interest in disorders of
human communication, particularly those of the elderly.

Peggy David, M.S.W.
Social Worker
Virginia Regional Spinal Cord Injury Project
University of Virginia
Charlottesville, Virginia 22908
After receiving a baccalaureate degree at the University of
Cincinnati, she obtained a master's degree in medical social
work from Washington University in St. Louis, Missouri. As
a spinal cord injury project social worker, she has presented
lectures at various schools and hospitals on the psychosocial
and sexual needs of the disabled.

Marilyn Donato, R.D.
Consulting Dietitian
3707 Alton Rd., S.W.
Roanoke, Virginia 24014
A member of the American Dietetic Association, Mrs. Donato
is a pioneer in establishing a private practice in nutrition
counseling for patients and in providing consultation in
diet therapy to area physicians. She is a board member of
the Roanoke Sub-Area Council of the Southwestern Virginia
Health Systems Agency, a food editor of several Philippine-

American newspapers, and the author of "Philipppine Cooking
in America." Mrs. Donato is experienced in geratric
rehabilitation, dietary needs of the long-term renal
dialysis patient, dietary care of the nursing home patient,
and is a booster for the Meals-on-Wheels program.

Philip S. Fogg, M.D.
Chief of Staff
Veterans Administration Medical Center
Salem, Virginia 24153
and
Assistant Professor of Behavioral Medicine and Psychiatry
University of Virginia School of Medicine
Dr. Fogg has served the Veterans Administration as a chief
of an ambulatory care service, as a chief of psychiatry, and
now as a chief of staff, where he is expressing his particular concern for the problems of older, indigent patients by
helping them obtain humane care after hospitalization for
acute illness.

James C. Folsom, M.D.
Director
Institute for Crippled and Disabled (ICD) Rehabilitation and
Research Center
340 E. 24th St.
New York, New York 10010
Dr. Folsom is the Clinical Professor of Psychiatry at New
York University (N.Y.U.) Medical Center and Clinical Pro-
fessor of Rehabilitation Counseling at the N.Y.U. School
of Education, Health, Nursing and Arts Professions. He
started the first rehabilitation bed service for geriatric
patients in the Veterans Administration system in Topeka,
Kansas, and established the Reality Orientation Training
Program. For four years he was director of rehabilitation
medicine service in the V.A. Central Office, Washington,
D.C. Presently, as director of the oldest vocationally
oriented rehabilitation facility in the United States, he
is establishing a special day care program designed to
prevent hospitalization of confused, disoriented, elderly
individuals.

Ralph Goldman, M.D.
Assistant Chief Medical Director for Extended Care
Department of Medicine and Surgery
Veterans Administration Hospital, Dr. Goldman became
Associate Professor of Medicine at the University of
California at Los Angeles, with responsibility for
geriatrics and nephrology. Active in geriatrics, he was
a consultant to two White House Conferences on Aging,

chairman of the American clinical section of two Internationa
Congresses of Gerontology, chairman of the clinical section
of 1966 Gerontological Society, and president of the western
division of the American Geriatric Society. A professor of
medicine and assistant dean for allied health professions,
he was appointed assistant chief medical director for
extended care with responsibility for geriatrics at the
Veterans Administration Central Office in May 1977.

Harold B. Haley, M.D.
Associate Dean, Roanoke
and Professor of Surgery
University of Virginia School of Medicine
Roanoke, Virginia 24014
Dr. Haley coordinates the University of Virginia education
programs at Roanoke Memorial Hospitals, the Community
Hospital of Roanoke Valley and the Veterans Administration
Medical Center in Salem. He is a director of the Southwest
Virginia Health Systems Agency. Research interests include
physician attitudes and care of patients, problems in care
of cancer patients, and medical anthropology.

Mary Kate House, M.A.
4 Mile Road
R. R. #5
Richmond, Kentucky 40475
Mrs. House attended the George Peabody College for Teachers
in Hashville, Tennessee, and received her M.A. from Eastern
Kentucky University, Richmond, Kentucky. She lives on a
tobacco and cattle farm near Richmond with her husband, two
teenage sons, a 26-year-old married daughter and her twenty-
month-old grandson. A former teacher of English, French and
history, Mrs. House writes articles collects local ghost
and humorous stories, and goes horseback riding when she is
not caring for her family.

Patricia A. Keenan
Administrative Assistant
University of Virginia School of Medicine
Roanoke, Virginia 24014
Patricia A. Keenan attended Chicago's Loyola University
and Mundelein College where she majored in English and
History. Since 1959 she has been involved with research
and editing in areas of hypertension, physician attitudes,
patient care, cancer patients, and anthropology, first at
Stritch School of Medicine at Loyola University, and then
at the University of Virginia School of Medicine from 1972
to the present time.
    From 1969-72 she was Director of Admissions at the
Medical College of Ohio Toledo.

Perry F. Kendig, Ph. D.
Professor Emeritus of English and former President of
Roanoke College
Salem, Virginia 24153
A graduate of Franklin and Marshall College, he obtained
an A.M. and a Ph.D. at the University of Pennsylvania.
He served as dean of students and head of the English
department of Muhlenberg College. After coming to Roanoke
College as Dean and Professor of English in 1952, he became
President and Professor of English in 1963, retiring as
Professor Emeritus and President in 1975. He is a member
of the Governor's Bi-racial Citizens Advisory/Monitoring
Committee, various professional and ornithological associations, and scientific and community service boards. He has
served as president of the Virginia Foundation for Independent Colleges, the Association of Virginia Colleges, and
the Council of Lutheran Church in American Colleges.

Linda Kessinger, M.S.
Rehabilitation Counselor
Virginia Regional Spinal Cord Injury Project
University of Virginia
Charlottesville, Virginia 22908
Ms. Kessinger obtained her master's degree in rehabilitation
at West Virginia University. She served as a psychology
intern for the U.S. Department of Justice, and on the
Psychology Service, Veterans Administration Hospital,
Clarksburg, West Virginia, before coming to Woodrow Wilson
Rehabilitation Center, Fishersville, Virginia, where she
manages a caseload of twenty spinal cord injured individuals
in intermediate care.

Norman J. Knorr, M.D.
Dean
University of Virginia School of Medicine
Charlottesville, Virginia 22908
After receiving his M.D. from George Washington University
School of Medicine, Dr. Knorr trained in psychiatry at the
University of Maryland and John Hopkins Hospital, becoming
an assistant professor of psychiatry and plastic surgery in
1966. At the University of Virginia Hospital and Medical
Center Dr. Knorr became Director, Psychiatric Liaison-
Consultation Services in 1972, and Associate Dean in 1973,
before assuming his present position. Dr. Knorr is also a
professor of behavioral medicine and psychiatry and professor
of plastic surgery. He has published extensively in the
area of the psychiatric aspects of trauma and reconstructive
surgery.

Margaret E. Kuhn
National Convenor
Gray Panthers
6342 Greene Street
Philadelphia, Pennsylvania 19144
Maggie Kuhn worked for many years as associate secretary in
the United Presbyterian Office of Church and Society,
retiring by mandate in 1970 from her position as coordinator
of programs in the division of church and race. She
organized the Gray Panthers who "affirm aging as a life
spanning process of growth and development from birth to
death. Old age is an integral part of the whole, bringing
fulfillment and self-actualization." This self-actualized
lady has just published her latest book, "Maggie Kuhn on
Aging," and travels over 100,000 in the course of a year
conducting workshops and speaking about "the people who
celebrate growing up and growing old."

Mary Elyn Lauth, M.S.W.
Executive Director
New River Valley Agency on Aging
Pulaski, Virginia 24301
Recently, as a Levi Strauss fellow at the Ethel Percy Andrus
Gerontology Center, University of Southern California, Mrs.
Lauth engaged in intensive study of alternatives to institu-
tionalization and case management for the frail and elderly.
She administers a variety of programs for the 15,000 elderly
residents of a four-county rural area in southwestern
Virginia.

Richard W. Lindsay, M.D.
Associate Professor of Internal Medicine and Family Practice
University of Virginia School of Medicine
Charlottesville, Virginia 22908
After obtaining his medical degree from New York Medical
College, Dr. Lindsay trained in internal medicine at the
University of Virginia. He developed their Family Practice
Training Program. In 1977 Dr. Lindsay was appointed head
of the new division of geriatrics of the department of
internal medicine and initiated the first formal course in
geriatrics offered to medical students. He holds a grant
to study geriatric education in the U.S. and is developing
a geriatric evaluation center at the Blue Ridge Sanitorium.
Dr. Lindsay is a consultant in geriatrics at the Salem
Veterans Administration Medical Center. He recently received
a Geriatric Medicine Academic Award from the National
Institute on Aging. Dr. Lindsay is a member of the public
policy and the research and education committees of the
American Geriatrics Society.

Nancy L. Lohmann, Ph.D.
Associate Professor of Social Work
School of Social Work
West Virginia University
Morgantown, West Virginia   26506
Dr. Lohmann received a master's degree from the School of
Public Affairs, University of Minnesota, and a doctorate
in Social Welfare Administration, Policy, and Planning from
Brandeis University. Program director of the Appalachian
Gerontology Program, a multidisciplinary, university-wide
gerontological center, Dr. Lohmann's research concerns the
measurement of life satisfaction, morale, and adjustment.
She is particularly interested in the impact of institu-
tionalization on the social-psychological aspects of the
elderly individual, especially the rural elderly.

George L. Maddox, Ph.D.
Professor of Sociology
Director, Center for the Study of Aging and Human Development
Duke University Medical Center
Durham, North Carolina   27710
Educated at Millsaps College, Boston University, and Michigan
State University, Dr. Maddox received his Ph.D. in Sociology
in 1956. A past president of the Gerontological Society and
a founding member of the National Advisory Council, National
Institute on Aging as well as their consultant since 1975,
Dr. Maddox has also served as consultant on Alcohol Studies
at National Institute of Mental Health, and on the Advisory
Committee, White House Conference on Aging. He has written
extensively on the social aspects of later life, particularly
on adaptation to life-cycle events and on health care systems.

Nina G. Magier, M.D.
Staff Psychiatrist
Veterans Administration Medical Center
Salem, Virginia 24153
and
Assistant Professor of Psychiatry
University of Virginia School of Medicine
After studying philosophy in Warsaw, Dr. Magier obtained
her medical degree at the University of Vilno, Poland, in
1938. Following training and practice in pediatrics in
Poland and Germany, she was trained in psychiatry in Albany,
New York, and certified by the American Board of Psychiatry.
Dr. Magier has been concerned with geriatric medicine for
the past twenty years. She is consultant on Intermediate
Care Medicine at Veterans Administration Medical Center,
and a consultant in Geriatrics to Catawba Hospital.

Frank H. Mays, M.H.A.
Director
Southwest Virginia Health Systems Agency
Blacksburg, Virginia 24060
After receiving his undergraduate degree from the University
of Virginia and his master's in hospital administration from
the Medical College of Virginia, Mr. Mays obtained adminis-
trative residency training at the University of Virginia
and the Norfolk General Hospital. After seven years as
executive director of Roanoke Valley Health Services
Planning Council, he entered his present role. On a
statewide level, Mr. Mays is chairman of the Virginia
Health Interview Council and a member of the Virginia
Health Statistics Advisory Council.

Jeanne C. Miller, R.N., Ph.D.
Associate Professor
Chairman, Graduate Mental-Psychiatric Nursing Program
University of Virginia School of Nursing
Charlottesville, Virginia 22903
Dr. Miller received her Ph.D. degree in sociology from the
University of Nebraska in 1975. From 1976 to 1978 she was
research associate in gerontological nursing at Pennsylvania
State University, joining the University of Virginia in 1978.
Her primary concern is with the elderly, focusing upon
research on assessing abilities of the elderly for self-help
and mobilizing networks to assist the lederly in self-help
efforts. She is a consultant to the National Institute of
Mental Health.

T. Stuart Payne
Vice-President and General Manager
McVitty House, Inc.
Salem, Virginia 24153
Mr. Payne has been with McVitty House for fourteen years.
He helped develop and construct this unique institution for
elderly people, most of whom are poor. A leader in church
and community affairs, Mr. Payne is a former president of
the Virginia Nursing Home Association.

William E. Reefe, M.D.
Chief
Medical Service
Veterans Administration Medical Center
Salem, Virginia 24153
and
Professor of Internal Medicine
University of Virginia School of Medicine
After receiving his medical degree from Georgetown University
School of Medicine, Dr. Reefe trained in physical medicine
and rehabilitation in internal medicine with a subspecialty

in rheumatology. He was chief of rehabilitation medicine
and director of the nursing home and long-term care unit,
Veterans Administration Medical Center, Reno, Nevada. Dr.
Reefe was chief of medical service at the Veterans Administration Medical Center, Washington, D.C., before coming to
Salem, where he directs an active teaching program for
students and residents.

Sanford J. Ritchey, Ph.D.
Associate Dean
College of Home Economics
Virginia Polytechnic Institute and State University
(V.P.I. & S.U.)
Blacksburg, Virginia 24060
As director of the center of gerontology, V.P.I. & S.U., Dr.
Ritchey is responsible for the development of a multidis-
ciplinary effort concerned with teaching, research, and
service activities. He has had considerable experience in
human nutritional research, teaching, and academic adminis-
tration. Recent research projects have focused on the
elderly and the aging process.

Jorge Roman, M.D.
Chief, Nephrology Section
Medical Service
Veterans Administration Medical Center
Salem, Virginia 24153
and
Associate Professor of Internal Medicine
University of Virginia School of Medicine
After receiving his medical degree in Chile, Dr. Roman completed his training in internal medicine and a fellowship in
nephrology at the University of Virginia. Dr. Roman is renal
transplant coordinator for the Roanoke Valley and operates
the dialysis unit at the V.A.M.C. He has provided leader-
ship and training to several community-based dialysis centers
and conducts a training program for patients and their
families in home dialysis.

Roger A. Ruth, Ph.D.
Assistant Professor of Otolaryngology
University of Virginia School of Medicine
Charlottesville, Virginia 22908
Dr. Ruth received his doctorate from Ohio State University
and is currently director of the audiology division in the
Department of Otolaryngology and Maxillofacial Surgery at
the University of Virginia. Dr. Ruth has written extensively
on the physiology and pathophysiology of the human acoustic
reflex. In addition, he has had a special interest in
hearing problems of the aging patient, especially as they
relate to hearing aids and their value in presbyacusis.

Charles J. Schleupner, M.D.
Chief, Infectious Disease Section
Medical Service
Veterans Administration Medical Center
Salem, Virginia 24153
and
Assistant Professor of Internal Medicine
University of Virginia School of Medicine
Dr. Schleupner received his medical degree from the Univer-
sity of Maryland and trained in internal medicine and
infectious diseases at the University of Utah Medical Center.
Dr. Schleupner's research interests have included investiga-
tions into host defenses against viral infections, and the
effect of underlying disease and age upon these defense
mechanisms.

Maurice D. Schnell, M.D.
Professor, Department of Rehabilitation Medicine
and
Assistant Medical Director, Regional Rehabilitation Medicine
East Carolina University School of Medicine
Greenville, North Carolina 27834
Dr. Schnell received his medical degree, trained in Orthopedic Surgery, and received a fellowship in rheumatology and
rehabilitation at the University of Iowa. Later he received
a fellowship in rehabilitation medicine at Texas Institute
for Rehabilitation and Research, Houston. From 1966 to 1972
Dr. Schnell was an assistant professor in the department of
orthopedic surgery at the University of Iowa. From 1973 to
1978 he was an associate professor, department of orthopedics
and rehabilitation, director of rehabilitation medicine, and
medical director, rehabilitation engineering center, university of Virginia School of Medicine.

Eugene A. Stead, M.D.
Professor of Medicine
Chairman Emeritus, Department of Medicine
Duke University School of Medicine
Durham, North Carolina 27706
Retiring from the position of chairman of the department of
medicine at Duke in 1967, and this year from the position of
Medical Director, Methodist Retirement Home of Durham, he
continues to teach on the public and private wards of Duke
University Hospital, and at national and international con-
ferences on the problems of the aged. Because of his leader-
ship in medical education, Dr. Stead received the Abraham
Flexner Award of the Association of American Medical Colleges

R. Knight Steel, M.D.
Head, Division of Geriatrics
Boston University School of Medicine
Boston, Massachusetts 02115
A graduate of Yale University and Columbia College of
Physicians and Surgeons, Dr. Steel served six years on the
faculty of the University of Rochester Medical Center in
the Department of Medicine. At Boston University he is a
director of a three-year-old gerontology center that brings
together myriad university disciplines, which coordinate
activities to strengthen the health and welfare of
elderly persons.

Ralph J. Stoudt, Jr., Ph.D.
Associate Professor
Department of Speech Pathology and Audiology
University of Virginia
Charlottesville Virginia 22903
After receiving his doctorate in speech pathology from
the University of Michigan, he became assistant director
of the university's residential therapy program for
aphasic adults. He then served as chief pathologist at
the Bill Wilkerson Hearing and Speech Center, Nashville,
Tennessee, before moving to Charlottesville, where he
emphasizes language rehabilitation for aphasic adults.

David B. Walthall III, M.D.
Chief, Continuing Education Division
Academic Affairs Education Service
Veterans Administration Central Office
Washington, D.C. 20004
Dr Walthall practiced medicine for eight years in Dublin,
Virginia. He then joined the faculty of the Medical College
of Virginia, subsequently becoming assistant dean for con-
tinuing education. He helped to develop the quality
assurance program and introduced modern principles and
practices of adult education in several areas. In the
Veterans Administration Central Office, Dr. Walthall con-
centrates on overall continuing education and the six
Veterans Administration regional medical education centers.

Mary Opal Wolanin, M.P.A., R.N.
Geriatric Nursing Consultant
3855 Calle Ensenada
Tucson, Arizona 85700
Twenty years after graduating from the Kansas City General
Hospital School of Nursing, Mrs. Wolanin obtained her B.A.
and M.P.A. degrees from the University of Arizona and went
on to become associate professor of nursing and a research
associate. She retired as Associate Professor Emeritus in

1977. During the past ten years she has been a consultant
to many hospitals, nursing homes, retirement centers, and
public agencies in the western United States. Mrs. Wolanin
is a member of several learned societies and has written
papers, books, and monographs on rehabilitation, nursing,
gerontology, and other nursing practices, based on her
research in geriatrics. She is particularly interested in
the study of communication in the elderly and in dispelling
myths about the aging process.

Index